TREAT YOUR OWN BACK

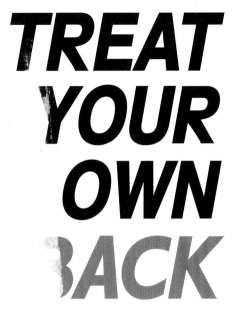

ROBIN McKENZIE O.B.E., F.C.S.P., F.N.Z.S.P.(Hon), DIP. M.T.

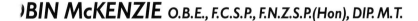

SPINAL PUBLICATIONS NEW ZEALAND LTD.

ISBN 0-9598049-2-7

First Published in 1980 by New Zealand University Press/Price Milburn

Second edition, published by Spinal Publications January, 1981

Third Edition   September, 1985
Fourth Edition   March, 1988
Fifth Edition   March, 1997

ACKNOWLEDGEMENT

My special thanks for assistance in the production of this edition must go to Joanne Moffat, my patient, loyal and untiring secretary.

I would also like to thank the following:

Office Furniture -	Economic Office Furniture, Wellington
Home Furniture -	Big Save Furniture, Wellington
Motor Vehicles -	Rutherford & Bond Toyota, Wellington

Robin McKenzie

One of the most remarkable facts of modern medicine is the variation in chronicity of backache in modern societies versus back problems in primitive societies. Physicians who care for patients in missionary hospitals and other facilities in the Third World report that chronic back and leg problems related to the lumbar discs are not common at all. Yet in our society with the benefit of modern care, backache is the most common musculoskeletal ailment. Indeed it is the most costly "disease" in the United States when we take account of disability costs in addition to the cost of medical care. What could be the explanation?

Inactivity, prolonged bedrest, the use of various electrical modalities such as diathermy and ultrasound, are all unknown modes of treatment in the primitive world. Activity is a necessity for all but the most woefully ill in these areas. In contrast, the customary care in western societies for the persistent back problem perhaps with associated leg pain usually starts with the comment by the physician or therapist: "Take it easy". Frequently this inactive care is associated with various modalities which are proposed to reduce muscle spasm and pain. Incidentally, there has never been a scientific study which demonstrates the effectiveness of such electrical gadgetry. Could there be a relationship between the inactivity of "modern" back care and the persistence of back problems in western societies today?

What are the most efficient and effective activities (exercise) to treat a backache? It has been demonstrated by research conducted at our own institution as well as others that an active treatment plan, including the special exercises for the back described in this book, is more likely to result in the resolution of a disc problem than inactive treatment. These McKenzie exercises are different than the usual programmes focused at muscle strengthening. These exercises are focused at improving the structure and metabolism of the soft tissues including the disc. The nice part about this active treatment is that we can do it for ourselves easily. It requires very little equipment. Ideally it is performed with the supervision of a trained therapist, but in general much of the treatment can be accomplished following a few basic guidelines as outlined in this book.

Thus, I am very pleased to recommend this volume by Robin McKenzie. It is a safe and reliable method to resolve back problems related to the injured disc. It has never caused harm to the patient. It is extremely inexpensive. For those very few patients who fail to improve on this method, specialized medical care can usually provide a clear-cut answer and solution.

With greater utilization of the methods advocated in this book, one can expect the health of the back to improve. In fact, we have good reason to think that the healthier back is less liable for repeat injury. Thus we really can treat our own backs.

Vert Mooney, MD,
Professor of Orthopaedics
UCSD OrthoMed Medical Director
University of California, San Diego
La Jolla, California, U.S.A.

ABOUT THE AUTHOR

Robin McKenzie was born in Auckland, New Zealand, in 1931. After attending Wairarapa College he enrolled in the New Zealand School of Physiotherapy, from which he graduated in 1952. Since 1953, when he commenced private practice in Wellington, New Zealand, he has specialised in the treatment of spinal disorders.

During the sixties Robin McKenzie developed his own examination and treatment methods and is now recognised internationally as an authority on the diagnosis and treatment of low back pain. He has lectured worldwide and to give some measure of the success of the system of treatment he has developed, his methods are now practised in North and South America, Eastern and Western Europe, Africa, the Middle East, Scandinavia, Asia, Australia and New Zealand. In the United States, there is evidence that the McKenzie method is the preferred treatment for back problems among physiotherapists.

The success of the McKenzie concept of treatment has attracted considerable interest from researchers in various parts of the world and it is one of the most researched treatment systems for back pain at the present time. Several research projects demonstrate the efficacy and importance of the system. In one of the more important studies by internationally renowned researchers from the University of Washington in the United States, it was shown that one month after completing treatment, patients receiving the McKenzie method improved to the same degree as patients receiving manipulation provided by chiropractors. More importantly, the patients treated by the McKenzie system had fewer treatments to achieve that improvement and 72% reported that in the event of recurrence they felt they could manage their own problem.

To ensure the orderly development of education and research into the methods devised by Robin McKenzie, doctors and physiotherapists involved in the teaching process formed the McKenzie Institute International in 1982 . The Institute is a non profit organisation with headquarters in New Zealand. Robin McKenzie was elected the first president.

Mr McKenzie has published in the New Zealand Medical Journal and contributed to many authoritative texts on back problems. He is the author of four books, "Treat Your Own Back", "Treat Your Own Neck" (which have been translated into seventeen languages), "The Lumbar Spine, Mechanical Diagnosis and Therapy", and "The Cervical and Thoracic Spine, Mechanical Diagnosis and Therapy".

The contributions Robin McKenzie has made to the understanding and treatment of spinal problems have been recognised both in New Zealand and internationally. In 1982 he was made an Honorary Life Member of the American Physical Therapy Association, "in recognition of distinguished and meritorious service to the art and science of physical therapy and to the welfare of mankind." In 1983 he was elected to membership of the International Society for the Study of the Lumbar Spine. In 1984 he was made a Fellow of the American Back Society, and in 1985 he was awarded an Honorary Fellowship of the New Zealand Society of Physiotherapists. In 1987 he was made an Honorary Life Member of the New Zealand Manipulative Therapists Association and in 1990 an Honorary Fellow of the Chartered Society of Physiotherapists in the United Kingdom. In the 1990 Queen's Birthday Honours, he was made an Officer of the Most Excellent Order of the British Empire.

CONTENTS

THE CHANCE DISCOVERY

In about 1956 in my clinic in Wellington, New Zealand, I observed by chance a remarkable event which has changed worldwide the nature of treatment administered for the alleviation of back pain. This serendipitous event led to the development of the theories and practice that have now become the hallmark of the McKenzie methods for the diagnosis and treatment of common painful back problems.

The chance observation arose from a sudden change in the condition of a patient whom we will call Mr Smith. Mr Smith had pain to the right of his low back, extending into the buttock and thigh as far as his knee. He had undergone the conventional treatment considered suitable for back pain in that era. After three weeks of heat and ultra sound his condition had not improved. He had difficulty standing upright, he could bend forwards, but could not bend backwards. I told him to undress and lie face down on the treatment table, the end of which had been raised for a previous patient. Without adjusting the table, and unnoticed by any of the clinical staff, he lay face down with his back arched and over-stretched for some five minutes. When I returned in order to commence his treatment, I was extremely concerned to find him lying in what at that time was considered to be a most damaging position. On enquiring as to his welfare, I was astounded to hear him say that this was the best he had been in three weeks. All pain had disappeared from his leg. Furthermore, the pain in the back had moved from the right side to the centre. In addition, he found he could now bend backwards without having severe pain.

When Mr Smith arose from the treatment table, he could stand upright and he remained improved with no recurrence of leg pain. I placed him in the same position the following day, and this resulted in complete resolution of the remaining symptoms.

The important point to remember about all this is that as Mr Smith lay in this position, his pain changed location and moved from the leg and right side of his back to the centre point just at the waistline. The movement of pain from the leg or buttocks to the middle of the back is now known worldwide as the "centralisation phenomenon."

We now know that when pain moves, as it did in the case of Mr Smith, our chances of helping you with the methods described in this book, are very good indeed.

Thanks to the chance observation with Mr Smith, the McKenzie system is now provided worldwide by thousands of physiotherapists, doctors and chiropractors treating patients with back pain.

CHAPTER 1

ABOUT THE PROBLEM

So you continue to have recurring problems with your back. The attacks are not getting less frequent and may be more disabling than previously. Or is it that you have a chronic problem that is not responding to physiotherapy, chiropractic or the medication prescribed by your doctor? Or have you had surgery that has failed to correct the problem? You can only be reading this book because all else has so far failed.

The majority of the one thousand patients I saw every year for thirty-five years, taught me that the only people who really needed my services were those with recurrent or chronic back problems. These patients also taught me that most of them could learn to manage their own problem once they knew what to do. Indeed, it became clear that by applying spinal manipulation or adjustment to all my patients, I was prevented from identifying those who required only exercise. By teaching all patients to perform exercises specifically tailored to suit their own problem, I learned to identify the few who did require manipulation or adjustment.

Once taught self-management, most patients with recurring problems will willingly shoulder the responsibility for their own care. At last there is light at the end of the tunnel!

Low back pain, which affects nearly every one of us at some stage of our active adult life, is one of the most common ailments afflicting mankind. It is described in many ways such as fibrositis, slipped disc,

1

lumbago, arthritis in the back, rheumatism; or, when it causes pain extending into the leg, sciatica.

To most people low back pain remains a mystery. It often starts without warning and for no obvious reason; it interferes with simple activities of living, moving about and getting a comfortable night's sleep; and then, just as unexpectedly, the pain subsides. When in acute pain we are usually unable to think clearly about our trouble and simply seek relief from the pain. On the other hand, as soon as we have recovered from an acute episode, most of us quickly forget our low back problems. Once we have developed recurrent low back pain, we cannot do anything else but seek assistance, time and again, to become painfree. Usually, due to a lack of knowledge and understanding, we are unable to deal with present symptoms ourselves and until now have had no way of preventing future low back problems.

The causes of most kinds of common low back problems are quite clear. First I will explain why low back pain may occur. Then I will suggest how you can avoid it; or, if at present you are having low back pain, how you may recover from it and what steps to take should it reappear.

The main point of this book is that the management of your back is **your responsibility**. Of course, you can call on people with particular skills - doctors, physiotherapists or chiropractors - for treatment but in the end **only you can really help yourself**. Self-treatment of low back pain is now widely accepted; it will be more effective in the long-term management of your low back problems than any other form of treatment.

Many publications set out to tell you how to look after your own back and you may well wonder why yet another one is now offered. The reason is that this is the first book to show you how to *put your back in* if you are unfortunate enough to have *put it out*; and in addition it shows you what steps you must take to avoid recurrence.

Our research has told us that few people buy this book for first time problems with their back. This book provides the most benefit for people with recurring and chronic problems. Our research also tells us that somewhere between sixty and seventy-five percent of the population who have back pain once, will experience recurrence or chronicity.

If you have developed low back pain for the first time you should consult a health care professional such as your family doctor, a specialist physiotherapist, or chiropractor. You should also seek advice if there are complications to your low back pain: for example if you have constant pain which is referred into your leg all the way to your foot; if you have numbness or weak muscles; if, in addition to the back pain, you feel unwell. All these circumstances indicate the need to consult a health professional.

The McKenzie Institute International has now provided education and training in the McKenzie methods to over 20,000 physiotherapists, chiropractors and doctors worldwide. Should the methods described in this book fail to give you sufficient relief from your problem you should consult a health provider trained in the

McKenzie system. Very often a one-on-one session with such an expert will clarify the nature of the problem and the steps you must take to resolve it.

To obtain the names of Credentialed Members or Associates of the McKenzie Institute, see the Directory included at the back of the book.

CHAPTER TWO

THE LOW BACK OR LUMBAR SPINE

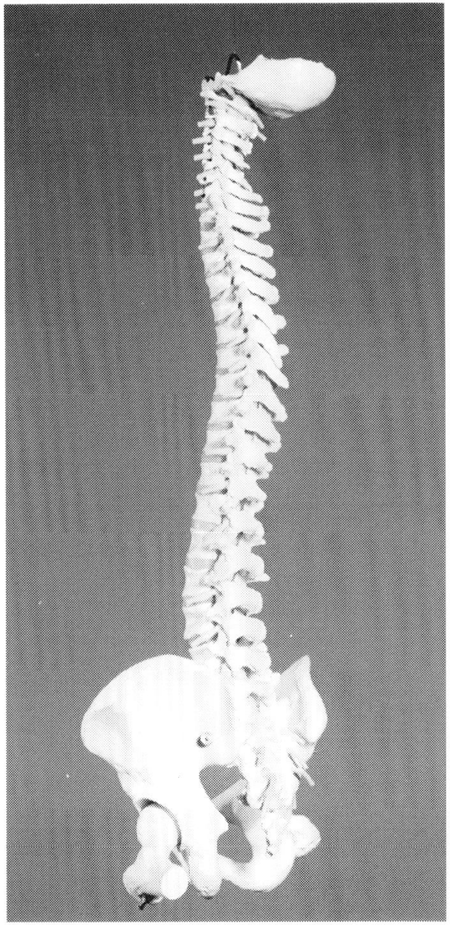

THE SPINE

If we look at the human backbone or spine, (*Fig.2.1*) we can see that the vertebrae rest upon one another similarly to a stack of cotton spools (*Fig.2.2*).

The spine is divided into regions. There are seven vertebrae in the cervical region, (neck), twelve vertebrae in the thoracic region, (upper back), and five vertebrae in the lumbar region (lower back). (*Fig.2:1*). Beneath the lumbar vertebrae are found the sacrum and the coccyx. It is the lower back or lumbar and sacral regions that concerns us most in this book.

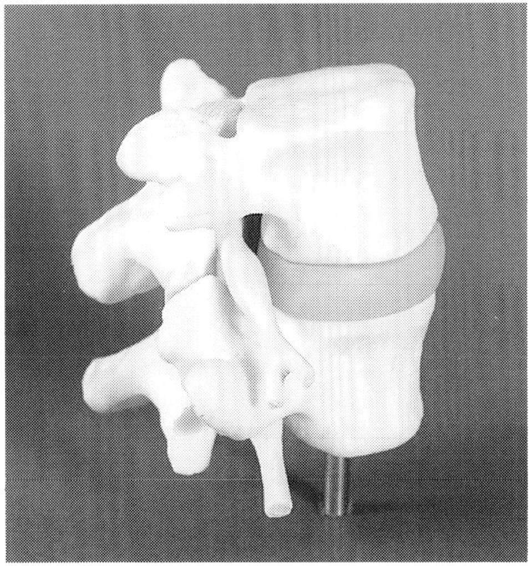

Fig 2.1 The human spine viewed from side and facing left.

Fig 2.2 Vertebrae similar to a stack of cotton spools

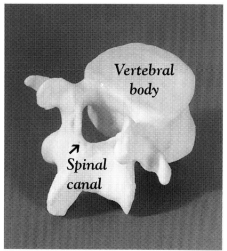

Vertebral body

Spinal canal

Fig 2.3

Each vertebra has a solid part in front, the vertebral body, and a hole in the back (*Fig.2:3*). When lined up as in the spinal column, these holes form the spinal canal. This canal serves as a protected passageway for the bundle of nerves which extends from head to pelvis - the spinal cord.

Special cartilages, called the discs, separate the vertebrae. The discs are located between the vertebral bodies just in front of the spinal cord (*Fig.2:2*). Each disc consists of a soft semi-fluid centre part, the nucleus, which is surrounded and held together by a cartilage ring, the annulus or annular ligament. The discs are similar to rubber washers and act as shock absorbers. They are able to alter their shape, thus allowing movement of one vertebra on another and of the back as a whole.

The vertebrae and discs are linked by a series of joints to form the lumbar spine or low back. Each joint is held together by its surrounding soft tissues - that is, a capsule reinforced by ligaments. Ligaments can be likened to the stays that hold a mast in place on a sailing ship. If a stay were to give way, the mast will likely fall when subjected to extra strains.

Muscles lie over one or more joints of the low back and may extend upwards to the trunk and downwards to the pelvis. At both ends each muscle changes into a tendon by which it attaches itself to different bones. When a muscle contracts it causes movement in one or more joints.

Between each two vertebrae there is a small opening on either side through which a nerve leaves the spinal canal, the right and left spinal nerve (*Fig.2:4*). Amongst other tasks the spinal nerves supply our muscles with power and our skin with sensation. In other words, it is through the nerves that we can

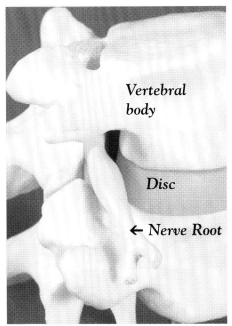

Vertebral body

Disc

← *Nerve Root*

Fig 2.4

move ourselves and feel temperature, pressure and pain. The nerves are really part of our alarm system: pain is the warning that some structure is about to be damaged or has already sustained some damage.

In the lower part of the spine some of these nerves combine on each side to form the right and left sciatic nerve. The sciatic nerves service our legs and when compressed or irritated they may cause pain in the leg which often extends below the knee. This is then called sciatica.

FUNCTIONS OF THE LUMBAR SPINE

In animals that walk on all fours the weight of their body is distributed evenly by their four legs. Most of the time the spine is held in a more or less horizontal position and the compressive forces that exist in upright man do not occur.

In human beings the spine is held in a more or less vertical position, at least during waking and working hours. When we are upright, the lumbar spine bears the compressive weight of the body above it, transmits this weight to the pelvis when sitting and to the feet when standing, walking and running. Thus the lumbar spine, providing a flexible connection between the upper and lower half of the body, protects the spinal cord and also has a greater function in weight bearing. In the evolution of the horizontal-spine posture of animals to the vertical-spine posture of man the discs between the vertebrae have adapted to support heavier weights. In addition the spinal column has developed a series of curves that ingeniously allow for better shock absorption and flexibility.

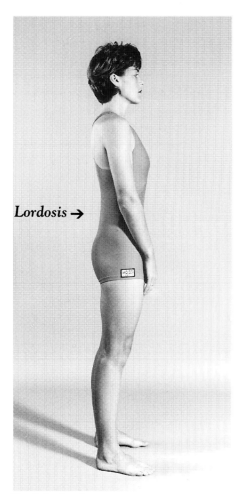

Lordosis →

Fig 2.5   Lordosis

NATURAL POSTURE

The side view of the human body in the standing position (*Fig.2:5*) shows that there is an inward curve in the small of the back just above the pelvis. This hollow in the low back is called the lumbar lordosis. The lumbar lordosis is a natural feature of the lumbar spine in all humans, having been formed during the evolutionary process. Our understanding of the function of the lumbar lordosis in an important feature of this book.

When standing upright the lordosis is naturally present, though it varies from person to person. The lordosis is lost whenever the low back is rounded and this usually occurs during sitting and bending forwards. If the lordosis is lost often and for long enough periods, then low back problems may develop. The ligamentous stays become fatigued or overstretched, and may give way, resulting in another painful episode!

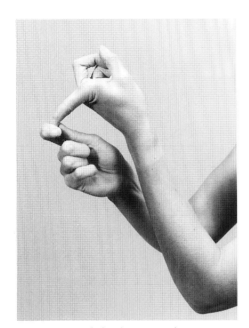

Fig 2.6   Bend the finger until
you feel the strain

MECHANICAL PAIN

This section on mechanical pain is very important as it explains exactly why you hurt when you do. If you take the time to well understand this section of the book, you will be more than halfway towards solving your problems. Our research has found that the better the patient understands the problem, the better will be the results of self-treatment.

Pain of mechanical origin occurs when the joint between two bones has been placed in a position that overstretches the surrounding ligaments and other soft tissues. This is true for mechanical pain in any joint of the body, including the spine. To help you understand how easily some mechanical pains can be produced, you may like to try a simple experiment.

Firstly, bend one finger backwards, as shown in *Fig.2:6*. Bend the finger until you feel a **strain**. If you cause the finger to remain in this strained position, you will initially feel minor discomfort only but, as time passes, **pain** will **eventually** develop. In some cases, pain caused by prolonged stretching may take as much as an hour to appear.

Try the experiment once more, but now keep bending the finger past the point of **strain** until you feel **pain**. The sensation of pain is **immediate**. You have overstretched, and your pain warning system is telling you that to continue movement in that particular direction will cause **damage**.

Should you ignore the warning and continue to overstretch, **damage** will occur. Of course the pain warning tells you to stop overstretching and when you do so the pain ceases immediately. No damage will have occurred to your finger and the pain will have gone.

No lasting problems will arise from this short-lived strain providing you take note of the pain warning system.

If you fail to heed the warning and keep the finger in the overstretched position, the ligaments and surrounding soft tissues that hold the joint together will be **torn**. This tearing will result in an ache which continues even when you stop overstretching. The pain will continue even when the finger is at rest. The pain will increase with movement and reduce at rest but it will not cease until some healing has occurred. Healing may take several days but will be prolonged if, every day, you continue to apply the same strains to the finger.

MECHANICAL LOW BACK PAIN

If an engineer were to examine which area in the back is subjected mostly to mechanical stress, he would conclude that most strain must be placed on that part of the spine which is located just above its junction with the pelvis. This conclusion is correct for statistics show that back problems arise more often in the low back than in any other part of the spine.

Low back pain is not caused by draughts, chills, or the weather. It was once believed that these weather related phenomena were responsible for back and neck pains. Today our understanding is better, and it is generally agreed by specialists that most backache is caused by mechanical strains, similar to those described in the previous section.

It is often thought that low back pain is caused by strained muscles. Muscles, which are the source of power and cause movement, can indeed be overstretched or injured. This requires a considerable amount of force and does not often happen. Moreover, muscles usually heal very rapidly and seldom cause pain lasting for more than a week or two. On the other hand, whenever the impact of the injuring force is severe enough to affect the muscles, the underlying soft tissues and ligaments will be damaged as well. In fact, usually these tissues are damaged long before the muscles.

Most low back pain is caused by prolonged overstretching of ligaments and other surrounding soft tissues. Just as pain arises in the overstretched finger as I have described above, pain can also arise in the lower back when ligaments in this region are overstretched. Pain produced by overstretching in this manner is **very** common and arises particularly when we develop poor postural habits. Whenever we remain in a relaxed position, be it standing, sitting, or lying, prolonged overstretching can easily occur.

When pain arises because we have allowed our posture to slouch, it is really our own fault and we have no one to blame but ourselves. This type of strain is easily avoided and once we have been properly educated, the prevention of pain produced in this manner becomes our responsibility.

However, mechanical pain may also be caused by overstretching of such severity that some tissues are actually **damaged**. Overstretching causing **damage** may occur when an outside force places an excessive strain on the low back. For example, this type of strain can occur due to a fall while playing tennis, or from a contact sport such as football where severe forces develop when players are tackled. Lifting excessive weights is also likely to cause overstretching and damage to the supporting ligaments of the spinal joints. These types of injury cannot easily be avoided as they occur unexpectedly and without warning signs.

2

When soft tissues surrounding a joint are overstretched it is usually the ligaments that first give rise to pain. When the spinal joints are considered, there are additional factors, for the surrounding ligaments are also the retaining walls for the soft discs that act as shock absorbers between the vertebrae. Overstretching of these will, under certain circumstances, affect the discs. This may significantly influence or alter the intensity of the pain that you have, the distribution of the pain you feel, and the behaviour of the pain, which may be made better or worse by certain movements or positions.

Complications of another sort arise when the ligament surrounding the disc is injured to such an extent that the disc loses its ability to absorb shock and its outer wall becomes weakened. This allows the soft inside of the disc to bulge outwards and, in extreme cases, to burst through the outer ligament, which may cause severe pain. When the disc bulges far enough backwards, it may press painfully on the sciatic nerve. This can cause some of the pains or other symptoms (numbness, sensation of pins and needles, weakness) that may be felt well away from the source of the trouble, for example in the lower leg or foot.

Should the soft inside of the disc bulge excessively, the disc may become severely distorted. This will cause the vertebrae to tilt forward or to one side and prevent the vertebrae from lining up properly during movement. In this case some movements will be blocked partially or completely and any movement may cause severe pain. This is the reason why some people with severe back pain are forced to stand with the trunk off-centre or bent forward. Those of you who experience a sudden onset of pain and following this are unable to straighten up or move the back properly, are likely to have some bulging of the soft disc material. This need not be a cause for alarm.

The exercises, described in this book, are carefully designed to reduce any disturbance of this nature.

Once soft tissues are damaged, pain will be felt until healing is complete and function is fully restored. It is important that during the healing process you avoid movements that pull the healing surfaces apart. For instance, if you have overstretched ligaments of the lower back by bending forward, it is likely that any repetition of this movement will continue to open and separate the healing tissues and this will further delay the repair of the damage. If, on the other hand, you avoid bending forwards and instead keep a hollow in the lower back, the damaged surfaces will remain together and healing will not be interrupted.

It is difficult perhaps to visualise this process occurring in the lower back. Using the finger once more as an example may help your understanding. Let us imagine that you have accidentally cut across the back of your knuckle with a sharp instrument. If you were to bend the injured finger joint every day, you would open up the wound and delay recovery. However by keeping the finger straight for about a week, you would allow the healing surfaces to remain together and complete healing would result. You could then commence bending the finger without risking any further damage. The same strategy works for the problems arising in the lower back.

When tissues heal they form scar tissue. Scar tissue is less elastic than normal tissue and tends to shorten over time. If shortening occurs, movement may stretch the scars and produce pain. Unless appropriate exercises are performed to restore normal flexibility, the healed tissue may produce a continuous source of back pain and/or stiffness. Such problems can persist for years. Even though the original damage is repaired, the scar itself restricts movement and causes pain when stretched.

WHERE IS THE PAIN FELT?

The sites of pain caused by low back problems vary from one person to another. In a first attack pain is usually felt in the centre of the back - at, or near the belt line (*Fig.2:7*), or just to one side (*Fig.2:8*) - and in general it subsides within a few days. In subsequent attacks pain may extend to the buttock (*Fig.2:9*); and later still to the back or outside of the thigh down to the knee (*Figs.2:10*), or below the knee down to the ankle or foot (*Figs.2:11*). Less often pain is felt in the front of the thigh down

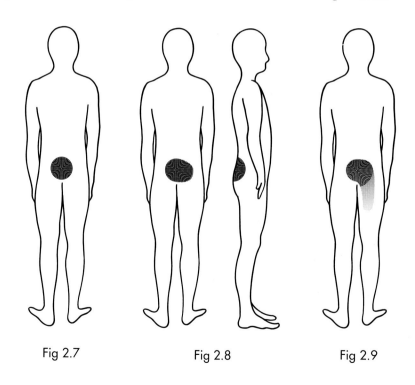

Fig 2.7   Fig 2.8   Fig 2.9

to the knee (*Fig.2:12*).

Pain may vary with movement or with position: the intensity of the pain can change, or the location of the pain can alter - for example, one movement may cause buttock pain, another may cause the pain to leave the buttock and appear in the low back.

If you have a very severe problem, in addition to low back pain you may experience significant numbness or muscular weakness in the lower leg.

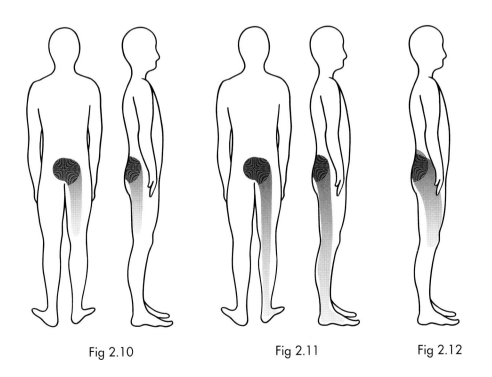

Fig 2.10   Fig 2.11   Fig 2.12

WHO CAN PERFORM SELF-TREATMENT?

Most people will benefit from the advice given in this book and can commence the exercise programme, provided the recommended precautions are taken. Once you have started the exercises, carefully watch your pain pattern. If your pains were worsening before you started the exercises and they do not subside after the first two days, you should seek advice from your health professional. Similarly, if your symptoms consistently increase immediately following the exercises and you remain worse over the following two days, you should discontinue the exercises and seek advice from your health provider.

In any of the following situations you should not commence the exercise programme without first consulting your health professional:

- *If you have severe pain in the leg below the knee and experience sensations of weakness, numbness or pins and needles in foot and toes.*
- *If you have developed low back problems following a recent severe accident.*
- *If, following a recent severe episode of low back pain, you have developed bladder problems.*
- *If you are feeling generally unwell in conjunction with this attack of low back pain.*

To help you to determine whether you can treat your low back pain successfully without further assistance, you should answer the following questions:

- *Are there periods in the day when you have no pain? Even ten minutes?*
- *Is the pain confined to areas above the knee?*
- *Are you generally worse when sitting for prolonged periods or on rising from the sitting position?*

- *Are you generally worse during or right after prolonged bending or stooping as in bedmaking, vacuuming, ironing, gardening or concreting?*
- *Are you generally worse when getting up in the morning, but improve after about half an hour?*
- *Are you generally worse when inactive and better when on the move?*
- *Are you generally better when walking?*
- *Are you generally better when lying face down? When testing this you may feel worse for the first few minutes after which time the pain subsides: in this case the answer to the question is yes.*
- *Have you had several episodes of low back pain over the past months or years?*

If you have answered *yes* to all the questions, you are an ideal candidate for the self-treatment programme outlined in this book.

If you have answered *yes* to four or more questions, your chances to benefit from self-treatment are good and you should commence the programme.If you have answered *yes* to only three or less questions, then some form of specialised treatment may be required and you should consult a health provider trained or credentialed in the McKenzie system.

It may be the case that at present the distortion in the affected joint is too great to be reduced effectively by self-treatment only. Special procedures such as manipulation or REPEX as provided by a credentialed therapist may be required. At a later stage, once the severe or acute pain has subsided, you will be advised as to which sequence of exercise is best for you.

To obtain the names of Credentialed Members or Associates of the McKenzie Institute, see the Directory included at the back of the book.

3

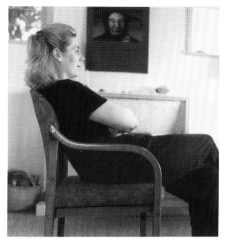

Fig 3.1   Poor seating position

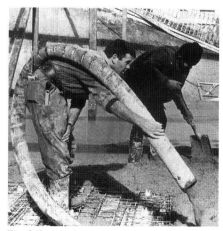

Fig 3.2   Awkward bending position

CHAPTER 3

COMMON CAUSES OF LOW BACK PAIN

POSTURAL CAUSES

The most common cause of low back pain is postural stress. Thus low back pain is frequently brought on by sitting for a long time in a poor position (*Fig.3:1*); or prolonged bending in bad working positions (*Fig.3:2*); heavy lifting (*Fig.3:3*); and standing (*Fig.3:4*) and lying for a long time in a poor position. When you look carefully at these photos, you will see that the low back is rounded and the lordosis has disappeared.

Unfortunately many people lose the lordosis much of the time and seldom or never increase it to its very maximum. If you reduce the lordosis for long periods at a time, year in, year out, and never properly restore it, you will eventually lose the ability to form the hollow. It is known that a flattened low back is frequently associated with chronic low back problems.

Most people naturally have a lordosis in the low back when they walk or run, and these activities often help to relieve low back pain. When we are standing the lordosis is naturally present but in some individuals, when the standing posture is maintained for a long time, the lordosis can become excessive and pain will be produced of a different nature than that occurring during prolonged bending.

Of all these postural stresses the poor sitting posture is by far the one most commonly at fault. A poor sitting posture in itself may produce low back pain. Once low back problems have developed, a poor sitting posture will perpetuate or worsen those problems.

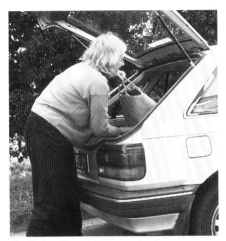

Fig 3.3   Poor lifting technique

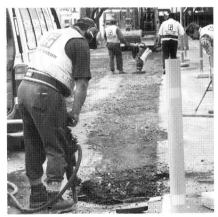

Fig 3.4   Standing in poor position

Poor standing postures and poor lying postures are also frequent causes of back pain. You may have already found that your back pain appears only if you stand for long periods or only after you get into bed. Pain that behaves in this way is frequently caused by poor posture alone. If this is the case, it is easily rectified.

The main theme of this chapter is that pain of postural origin will not occur if you avoid prolonged overstretching. Should pain develop, it is an almost certain indication that you have fallen into a poor position and immediate steps must be taken to correct your posture. Once the nature of your postural problem has been identified and you become aware of the steps you must take to correct it, you should not have to seek assistance whenever postural pain arises.

CONSEQUENCES OF POSTURAL NEGLECT

Some people who habitually adopt poor postures and remain unaware of the underlying cause, experience back pain throughout their lifetime simply because they were not in possession of the necessary information to correct the postural faults.

When pains of postural origin are first felt they are easily eliminated merely by correcting one's posture. As time passes, however, if uncorrected the habitual poor posture causes changes to the structure and shape of the joints, excessive wear occurs, and premature ageing of the joints is a consequence. The effects of poor posture in the long term, therefore, can be just as severe and harmful as the effects of injury.

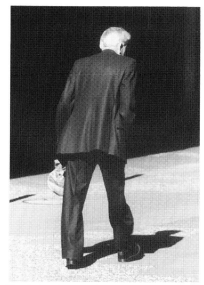

Fig 3.5   Stooped posture
in ageing

Those of us who allow poor posture to persist throughout our lifetime (*Fig.3:5*) become bent and stooped as the ageing process develops. When called upon to straighten and stand erect, we are unable to comply. When asked to turn the head, we are unable to do so. Our mobility is now so impaired we are considered by others to be affected by the normal ageing processes.

Deformities in the elderly are the visible effects of poor postural habit. There are secondary and sometimes severe consequences when these effects are transmitted to our body organs: the lungs are constricted and our breathing affected as the back becomes bent; the stomach and other internal organs are deprived of their correct support and may well be affected adversely.

It is my own opinion that the bent, stooped posture considered by many to be one of the inevitable consequences of ageing, is not at all inevitable and the time to commence preventive action is now. If we, but once a day, stand fully erect and bend fully backwards, we need never lose the ability to perform that action and therefore need never become bent, stooped and impaired in so many ways.

1. SITTING FOR PROLONGED PERIODS

Most people sitting for prolonged periods will eventually adopt a poor posture. When we sit in a certain position for a few minutes, the muscles that support our low back become tired, and relax. Our body sags and this results in the slouched sitting posture (*Fig.3:1*).

If we maintain a slouched sitting posture for long enough, it will

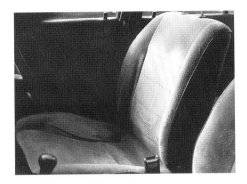

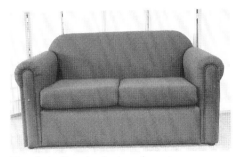

Figs 3.6 Poorly designed seating

cause overstretching of ligaments. Thus pain will arise when we have been sitting in **certain positions for prolonged periods**. Once the slouched sitting posture has become a habit and is maintained most of the time, it may also cause distortion of the discs contained in the vertebral joints. Once this occurs **movements as well as positions** will produce pain.

It follows that people with sedentary office jobs easily develop low back problems as they often sit with a rounded back for hours on end. If you are a sedentary worker, you may go through the following stages of gradually increasing back problems unless you take steps to rectify the cause. At first you may only experience discomfort in the low back while sitting for a prolonged period of time, or on arising from sitting. In this case the pain is caused by overstretching of soft tissues and it takes a few seconds for these tissues to recover. The pain at this stage is shortlived. At a later stage you will find that on standing up you have increased pain, and must walk carefully for a short distance before you can straighten up fully. Now it is likely that some distortion has occurred in one of the lumbar discs: prolonged sitting has led to minor distortion of the affected disc which needs a few minutes to recover. Eventually you may reach the stage when you frequently experience acute or agonising pain on standing and are unable to straighten up at all. In this case there is major distortion in the affected disc, which cannot regain its normal shape quickly enough to allow painfree movement. Whenever a movement is attempted, the disc bulge increases the strain on the already overstretched surrounding tissues. In addition, the disc bulge may pinch the sciatic nerve which may lead to pain and other symptoms in the leg.

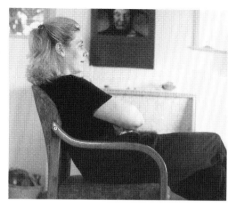

Fig 3.6   Poor sitting posture

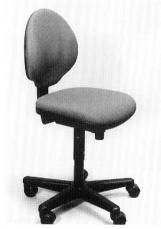

Fig 3.7   Well designed typist
or secretarial chair

ENVIRONMENTAL FACTORS

The design of transportation, commercial and domestic seating contributes to our poor postural habits. The chairs available rarely give adequate support to the low back and, unless a conscious effort is made to sit correctly, we are more or less forced to sit badly (*Fig.3:6*).

Ideally the back of all chairs should provide a lumbar support so that the lordosis, naturally present during standing, is also maintained while sitting (*Fig.3:7*). Unfortunately this support is rarely included. It is equally important that furniture in offices and factories is adapted to individual requirements. For example, if you are a desk worker you must make sure that the seat of your chair has the correct height. While sitting, your feet should rest flat on the floor and your thighs should remain horizontal without pressing on the seat. The desk itself must also be at the correct height; if the surface you lean on is too low, you will slouch forwards and lose the lordosis. Finally, arm rests must be positioned in such a way that, when using them, your shoulders are not unduly raised or lowered. Arm rests should also allow your chair to be pulled under the desk so that you can sit with your stomach held gently against the front of the desk. This will prevent you from leaning over and losing the lordosis while performing desk tasks. Until furniture designers understand the requirements of the human frame and work accordingly, we will continue to suffer from their neglect.

Although the poor design of furniture contributes to the development of low back problems, equal blame must be placed upon the individual who may use the chair improperly. If we do not know how to sit correctly, even the best chairs will not

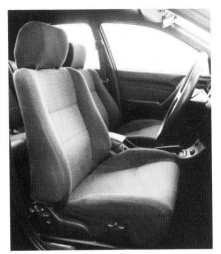

Fig 3.7   The McKenzie seat

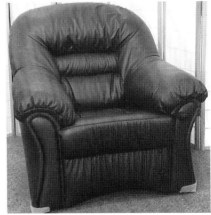

Fig 3.7

prevent us from slouching. On the other hand, once we have been instructed and the correct concepts have been instilled, poorly designed chairs will not have such a detrimental effect on our sitting posture.

Note: The McKenzie Institute in New Zealand was requested by the Toyota Car Company to provide expertise in the design of new seating for a range of their vehicles. From this cooperative venture has emerged a seat with outstanding qualities, combining spinal support and driver stability. The seat has met with universal customer approval especially when in use for extended journeys.

The McKenzie Institute has recently become involved in the design of domestic lounge furniture. It is the desire of the Institute to see well designed lounge furniture widely available and affordable.

SITTING CORRECTLY FOR PROLONGED PERIODS

If at the present time you have pain resulting from factors other than just poor posture, special exercises may need to be performed besides the postural correction. In this section I am only describing the exercises required to reduce postural stresses and obtain postural correction. The self-treatment exercises for relief of pain and increase of function will be dealt with in the next chapter.

So that you may **avoid the development of low back pain** due to prolonged poor sitting, it is necessary: (1) to sit correctly; and (2) to interrupt prolonged sitting at regular intervals.

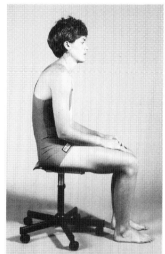

Fig 3.8   Extreme of slouched
sitting position

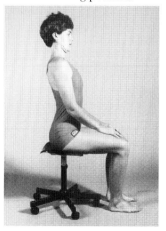

CORRECTION OF THE SITTING POSTURE

From now on you must pay a lot of attention to your sitting posture. You may have had the habit of sitting slouched for many years without low back pain, but once low back problems have developed you must no longer sit in the old way. The slouched posture will only perpetuate the overstretching and distortion within the joints.

In order to sit correctly you must first learn **how to form a lordosis** in the low back while sitting. Therefore you must become fully practised in the slouch-overcorrect procedure. Once you have achieved this, you must learn **how to maintain a lordosis** in the low back while sitting for prolonged periods.

HOW TO FORM A LORDOSIS

You must sit on a stool of chair-height or sideways on a kitchen chair. Allow yourself to slouch completely (*Fig.3:8*). Now you are ready to commence the slouch-overcorrect procedure.

Having relaxed for a few seconds in the slouched position, you should draw yourself up and accentuate the lordosis as far as possible (*Fig.3:9*). This is the extreme of the good sitting position. After holding yourself in this position for a few seconds, you should return to the fully relaxed position (*Fig.3:8*). The movement from the slouched to the upright sitting position should be done in such a way that you move rhythmically from the extreme of the bad to the extreme of the good sitting posture. The exercise must be performed

Fig 3.9   Accentuating the lordosis

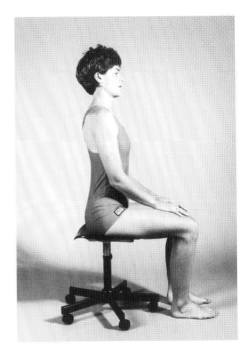

Fig 3.10   Extreme of good sitting
position - less strain creates
correct sitting posture

ten to fifteen times per session and the sessions are to be repeated three times per day, preferably morning, noon and evening. In addition you should do this exercise whenever pain arises as a result of sitting poorly. Each time you repeat this movement cycle you must make sure that movement is performed to the **maximum possible degree, especially towards the extreme of the good position**.

MAINTENANCE OF THE LORDOSIS

You have just learned how to find the **extreme of the good sitting posture.** It is not possible to sit in this way for long periods as it is a position of considerable strain and if maintained for excessive periods could actually cause pain. To sit comfortably and correctly you must sit short of the extreme good posture. To find this position you must first sit with your low back in extreme lordosis (*Fig.3:9*) and then release the last ten percent of the lordosis strain, taking care to ensure that you do not allow the low back to flatten (*Fig.3:10*). Now you have reached the correct sitting posture which can be maintained for any length of time. When sitting like this you maintain the lordosis in the low back with your own muscular effort; it requires constant attention and constant effort and you cannot fully relax. Whenever you sit in a seat **without a back-rest**, you must sit in this way.

THE LUMBAR ROLL

As few seats or chairs provide adequate support for the lower back, a portable lumbar roll is essential equipment for people with ongoing back problems. When sitting on a seat **with a back-rest** (supported sitting) a lumbar roll will facilitate the maintenance of a correct lordosis and posture.

A lumbar roll is a support specially designed for the low back (*Fig.3.11*). Without this support the low back will slouch whenever you are distracted or cease to concentrate on anything other than holding the lordosis actively with your own muscles - for example when talking, reading, writing, watching television or driving your car. To counteract this slouching you must place a lumbar roll in the small of your back at the level of your beltline whenever you sit in an easy chair (*Fig.3.12*), car (*Fig.3:13*) or office chair (*Fig.3.14*).

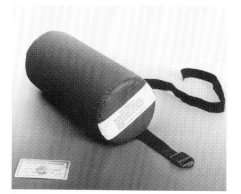

Fig 3.11   Lumbar roll

(You may purchase a lumbar roll specifically made for the purpose from the agents listed on the back cover of this book. You will need to supply them with your waist measurement and advise them how much you weigh.)

The lumbar roll should be no more than four to five inches (10-13 cm) in diameter before being compressed and should be moderately filled with foam so that under compression its diameter reduces to about one and a half inches (4 cm). A cushion does not serve the same purpose as it has the wrong shape and

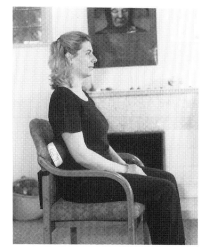

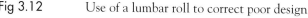

Fig 3.12   Use of a lumbar roll to correct poor design   Fig 3.13

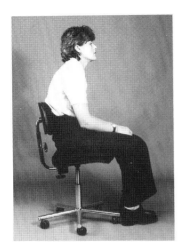

Fig 3.14

does not provide adequate pressure at the precise level of the low back. A regular cushion should not be relied upon for long-term use but may be of some assistance in an emergency.

The aim of this part of the programme is first to restore the correct posture and then to maintain it. It may take up to a week of practice to master this fully. As a rule, pain of postural origin will decrease as your sitting posture improves and you will have no pain once you maintain the correct posture. The pain will readily recur in the first few weeks should you allow yourself to slouch while sitting. Eventually you will remain completely painfree even when you forget your posture; however, never again should you allow yourself to sit slouched for long periods.

When first starting these procedures to correct your sitting posture, you will experience some new pains. These are different from your original pain and may be felt in other places. New pains are the result of performing new exercises and maintaining new positions, they should be expected and will wear off in a few days, provided postural correction is continued on a regular basis. Once you have become used to sitting correctly you will enjoy it, and will soon notice the reduction or absence of pain and the improved comfort. From then on you will automatically choose chairs that allow you to sit correctly.

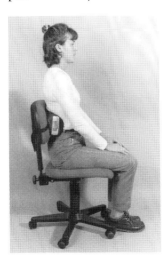

Fig 3.14 Use of a lumbar roll to correct poor design

RULE: When sitting for prolonged periods you must sit correctly with the low back in moderate lordosis. Whenever the seat has a back-rest you must use a lumbar roll to support the low back.

3

Note: In 1988 The McKenzie Institute commissioned a study to examine the effects of sitting with and without a lumbar roll. Patients in the group using the lumbar roll were required to use it at home, at the office, and whenever driving. The results showed conclusively that those patients using a portable lumbar roll whenever sitting, experienced much less pain than those not using a lumbar support.

Members of the McKenzie Institute worldwide are available to provide group education and instruction in the correction of posture in school children. The Institute has an educational video available to assist in this programme. For further information, contact a Member or Associate of the McKenzie Institute as listed in the Directory included at the back of the book.

REGULAR INTERRUPTION OF PROLONGED SITTING

Travelling for long distances by bus, car or airplane, especially when sitting in a cramped seat and without regular breaks which permit you to restore the lordosis, may cause a gradual and progressive attack of low back pain or may aggravate existing problems. Nearly everyone will be aware of some stiffness or discomfort in the low back after an uninterrupted car ride of a few hours. If you already have back problems, such a journey may be a risk situation for you. If you are the driver yourself, the risk is even greater.

In order to minimise the risks of prolonged sitting it is necessary that you interrupt sitting at regular intervals and **before pain starts**. For example, when undertaking long car journeys you should stop the car every hour, get out and bend backwards five or six times (see Exercise 4) and walk about for a few minutes. This will reduce the pressure within the discs and relieve the stresses on the surrounding tissues. As airlines continue to provide seating calculated to damage the human spine, you should, when flying long distances, regularly stand and walk up and down the aisle of the plane. This is not only important for the sake of your back but is also necessary to assist in the stimulation of the circulation in the legs. These are simple measures you can take that will significantly reduce the risk of another episode of back pain.

> **RULE:** When sitting for prolonged periods, regular interruption of the sitting posture is essential to prevent the onset of pain. This can be achieved by standing upright, bending backward five or six times, and walking about for a few minutes (See Exercise 4).

2. WORKING IN STOOPED POSITIONS

When standing with your back straight the stresses on discs and ligaments in your low back are considerably lower than when you stand with your back bent forwards. Many activities around the home may cause you to bend - for example gardening, vacuuming, bedmaking, etc (*Fig.3:15*). Occupations requiring prolonged stooped postures are abundant: assembly line workers, bricklayers, electricians, plumbers, carpenters, surgeons, nurses - the list goes on - are all required to bend forwards for prolonged periods every day. (*Fig.3:16*). While working in these bent positions, you are more likely to sustain back problems **in the first four or five hours of the day**.

In order to minimise the risks involved in prolonged forward bending you should interrupt the stooped position at regular intervals **before pain starts**. You should stand upright and bend backwards five or six times (see Exercise 4). This is very important if you have already developed low back problems

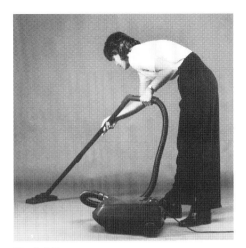

Fig 3.15

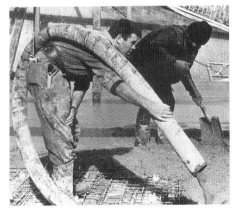

Fig 3.16   Prolonged stooped positions

3

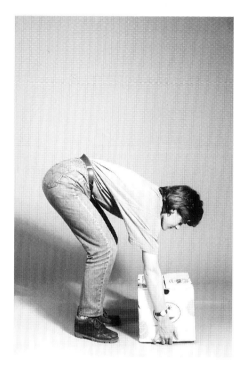

Fig 3.17   Poor lifting technique

caused by working in a stooped position. Regular interruption of the stooped position will correct any distortion that may occur in the discs and relieve the stresses on the surrounding tissues. When this is done **before pain starts**, it usually prevents the development of significant low back pain; and **remember, you are especially at risk in the first half of your day**, so make sure you always do everything correctly during this period.

> **RULE:** When working in a stooped position, regular interruption of the bent posture is essential to prevent the onset of pain. This can be achieved by standing upright and bending backwards five or six times. (See Exercise 4).

3. LIFTING

Lifting objects with your back rounded (*Fig.3:17*) has been found to raise the pressure in the discs to a much higher level than that existing when the weight is held with the body upright and the lordosis present. Just as back problems associated with bending seem to occur very frequently in the first four or five hours of the day, so it is with lifting; especially so if you are lifting repeatedly and frequently. If you use an incorrect lifting technique while lifting heavier objects, you may cause damage and, of course, sudden severe pain.

In order to minimise the risks involved in lifting you should always use the correct lifting technique (*Fig.3:17a-e*). You should stand upright and bend backwards five or six times immediately before and after lifting, especially when a single heavy lift is involved. If there are many objects to be lifted, you

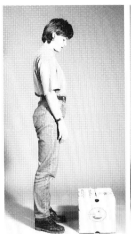
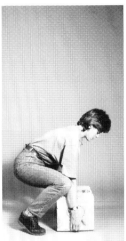

Fig 3.17a   Fig 3.17b

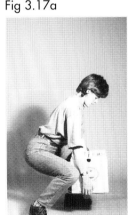
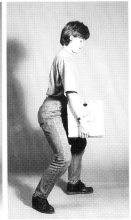
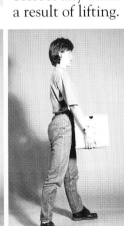

Fig 3.17c   Fig 3.17d   Fig 3.17e

should frequently interrupt the lifting and repeat the backwards bending exercise. By standing upright and bending backwards before lifting, you ensure that there is no distortion already present in the joints of the low back as you begin the lift. This is particularly important if you have been in a stooped position or have been sitting for a prolonged period immediately before you start lifting.

For example, many truck drivers after driving for prolonged periods are then called upon to remove heavy objects from the back of the truck. Removing heavy suitcases from the boot or trunk of the car immediately after a long ride is another example of this high risk situation. By standing upright and bending backwards a few times **before and after** lifting, you correct any distortion that may have developed in the joints as a result of lifting.

If at present you are suffering a bout of low back pain, especially when this is caused by lifting, it is best to completely avoid lifting for a few weeks so that healing of damaged tissues may take place. Should this not be possible, then you must at all times use the correct lifting technique and avoid lifting objects that are awkward to handle and heavier than thirty pounds (15 kg).

Once you have developed recurrent low back problems you should never again handle awkward or heavy objects by yourself, even though you may be completely painfree at the time of lifting. In addition, you should familiarise yourself with the correct lifting technique. After some practice at this, lifting correctly will become a habit.

CORRECT LIFTING TECHNIQUE

Throughout the lift you must attempt to retain the hollow in your low back (*Figs.3:17a b c d and e*). The lift should be applied by straightening the legs. Avoid using the back as a crane to lift the weight (*Fig.3:17*).

Correct lifting technique involves the following:

- *Stand close to the load, have a firm footing and a wide stance.*
- *Accentuate the lordosis.*
- *Bend your knees to go down to the load and keep your back straight.*
- *Get a secure grip and hold the load as close to you as possible.*
- *Lean back to stay in balance and lift the load by straightening the knees.*
- *Take a steady lift, do not jerk.*
- *When upright, shift your feet to turn and avoid twisting the low back.*

RULE: When lifting, you should apply the correct lifting technique. In addition, you should stand upright and bend backwards five or six times immediately before and after each heavy single lift and also at regular intervals during repeated lifting.

4. RELAXING AFTER VIGOROUS ACTIVITY

Over the years I have heard many people complain that they develop back pains after engaging in heavy activities such as concreting or gardening, and it is very easy to attribute such pains to these activities. But as so often occurs, after activity we sit and relax, very often collapsing slouched in a chair. Once we feel the onset of pain, we automatically attach the blame to the activity that we have just completed. We should, instead, consider the likelihood that the pain has commenced as a result of the posture we have since adopted.

If the activity itself had been responsible for the production of the pain, we would feel some discomfort or pain at the time of overstretching or injury, not an hour later when we are sitting relaxed. The joints of the spine after activity seem to undergo a loosening process and if we subsequently place ourselves in an unsupported position for prolonged periods, distortion within the joint readily occurs. **Thoroughly exercised joints** of the spine **distort easily** if they are placed in a **slouched position for long periods**.

RULE: After vigorous activity you should restore and accentuate the lordosis by standing upright and bending backwards five or six times. When you sit down to rest, you should maintain the lordosis and use a lumbar roll to avoid slouching.

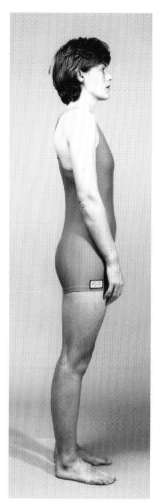

Fig 3.18

5. PROLONGED STANDING

Some people always get low back pain when standing in one place for a long time. Just as occurs when we are sitting for long periods, when we stand for long periods the muscles that support us tire and relax, allowing us to slouch. When we stand relaxed, however, the lordosis becomes excessive and the low back hangs in an extreme position. This is exactly the opposite position to that adopted by the spine when we sit slouched. It is not possible to stand in this way for long periods as the excessive lordosis is a position of strain. If your low back pain is produced during prolonged standing, you will find relief by correcting your standing posture.

CORRECTION OF THE STANDING POSTURE

To stand correctly you must hold your low back in a position of reduced lordosis. To find this position, you must first stand relaxed. Allow the chest to sag and the abdomen to protrude slightly; this will place the lower lumbar joints in an extreme lordosis . Now **reduce the lordosis by standing as tall as you can**. Lift the chest up, pull in your stomach muscles and tighten your buttocks (*Fig.3:18*). You have now reached the correct standing posture. When standing like this you reduce the lordosis with your own muscular effort. To begin with you will find it difficult to effectively hold this position, but with practice you can learn to stand in this new position for long periods without discomfort.

RULE: When standing for prolonged periods you must stand correctly. Stand tall. Do not allow your back to sag into extreme lordosis. Frequently stand tall.

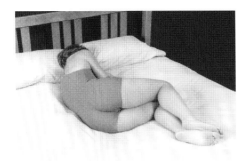

Fig 3.19

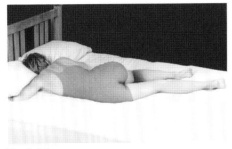

Fig 3.19

6. LYING AND RESTING

Some people have low back pain when they are lying resting in certain positions. A few people have low back pain only when they lie down. Many people with low back pain feel worse when they are lying down and dread the thought of another night with more back pain and less sleep.

If you have low back pain only when lying down, or if you regularly wake in the morning with a stiff and painful low back that was not painful the night before, there is likely to be something wrong with the surface on which you are lying or the position in which you sleep (*Fig.3:19*). It is a comparatively easy task to correct the surface on which you are lying, but rather difficult to influence the position you adopt while sleeping. Once you are asleep, you may regularly change your position or toss and turn. Unless a certain position causes so much discomfort that it wakes you, you have no real idea of the various positions you assume while sleeping.

Many people with back problems are told never to lie face down when in bed. There is no evidence whatsoever to suggest that this is harmful to the back. On the contrary, it may well be that your back ceases to be painful in the face down position. If you have not already discovered the effects of lying face down, you should experiment to see what effect this has on your problem the next time you experience pain while lying. Certainly there are some low back problems that are aggravated by lying in this way. If you have sciatica, lying face down is nearly always impossible.

3

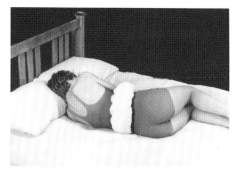

Fig 3.20

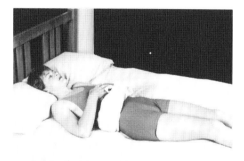

Fig 3.20

CORRECTION OF SURFACE

There are two simple ways in which you may be able to reduce strains on your low back caused by a faulty lying position:

The first and most important way is to lie with a supportive roll around your waist. The roll will support your low back as you rest and will prevent strain that can develop when you lie on your side or back.

You may purchase a lumbar night roll specifically made for the purpose from the agents listed at the back of this book. You will need to supply them with your waist measurement and advise them how much you weigh. Alternatively, you may substitute a rolled beach or bath towel. Fold the towel in half from end to end, then roll it from the side . This will create a roll of about three inches (7.5 cm) in diameter and three feet (90 cm) in length. Wind the roll around your waist, and fix it in front with a safety pin to ensure that it remains in place where you normally wear your belt; otherwise, should the roll move up or down during your sleep, it may actually increase your night pain. The measurements given above are merely a guide; lumbar supports need to fulfil individual requirements and each person must experiment for himself. You can follow the general rule that when you lie on your side, the roll should fill the natural hollow in the body contour between pelvis and rib cage; and when you lie on your back, the roll should support the low back in moderate lordosis (*Fig.3:20*).

The second way is to ensure that your mattress does not sag. The mattress itself should not be too hard; in fact, a soft mattress can be extremely comfortable provided it is placed on a firm support. To ensure that your mattress is supported on a firm hard surface, it is best to place it on the floor and spend three to four nights sleeping in this way to determine if this is the source of the problem. Avoid a bed with a wire base and use a solid base instead, with a rubber or innerspring mattress on top of it.

If you have tried these suggestions without benefit, you should consult a health provider trained in this specialty. Members or associates of the McKenzie Institute are well versed in the management of these problems. It may be that you require special advice regarding the surface on which you lie, or the posture you assume while sleeping. It may also be possible that you need special treatment for your low back problems.

7. COUGHING AND SNEEZING

Coughing and sneezing while you are bent forwards or sitting may cause a sudden attack of low back pain or aggravate existing back pain. If you sense the need to cough or sneeze, you should try to stand upright and bend backwards so that your low back is hollow at the moment you cough or sneeze. Should you not be able to stand up, then you must at least lean backwards and make the best possible lordosis.

CHAPTER 4

EXERCISES

GENERAL GUIDELINES AND PRECAUTIONS

The exercise programme consists of seven exercises: the first four exercises are extension exercises, the last three are flexion exercises. Extension means bending backwards and flexion means bending forwards.

The purpose of the exercises is to abolish pain and, where appropriate, **to restore normal function** - that is, to regain full mobility in the low back or as much movement as possible under the given circumstances. When you are exercising for pain relief, you should move to the edge of the pain or just into the pain, then release the pressure and return to the starting position; but when you are exercising to regain lost movement or for stiffness, you should try to obtain the maximum amount of movement, and to achieve this you may have to move well into the pain.

Postural correction and maintenance of the correct posture should always follow the exercises. Even when you no longer have low back pain and for the rest of your life, good postural habits are essential to prevent the recurrence of your problems

PAIN INTENSITY AND PAIN MOVEMENT
Read this section carefully

The exercises described in this book are not designed to strengthen the muscles of your back. We have found that if we can rid you of pain and return you to normal activity your strength will return in the normal course of events.

These exercises are designed to correct any distortion or bulging that may have developed in the joints of the lower back. By reducing the distortion or bulging of the intervertebral disc, we can in turn reduce the level of pain that you experience.

The exercises also identify for you any movements or postures that are likely to increase distortion in the joints thus delaying recovery. This will enable you to avoid damaging postures or activities in the future.There are three main effects that you may look for while performing the exercises. Firstly, the exercises may cause the symptoms to disappear. Secondly, they may cause an increase or decrease in the intensity of the pain that you experience. Finally they may cause the pain to move from where you usually feel it to some other location. In certain cases the symptoms will firstly change location, then they will reduce in intensity, and finally they will cease altogether.

The effects of exercise on the intensity or location of pain can sometimes be very rapid. It is possible to reduce the intensity or change the location of pain after completing as few as ten or twelve movements, and in some conditions the pain can completely disappear.

In order to determine whether the exercise programme is working effectively for you, it is very important that you observe closely any changes in the intensity or location of your pain. You may notice that pain, originally felt across the low back, to one side of the spine or in one buttock or thigh, moves towards the centre of the low back as a result of the exercise. In other words your pain **localises or centralises**.

Centralisation of pain (Fig.4:0) that occurs as you exercise is a good sign. If your pain moves to the midline of the spine and away from areas where it is usually felt, you are exercising correctly and this exercise programme is the correct one for you.

4

The centralisation of pain is the single most important guide you have in determining the correct exercises for your problem. The centralisation of pain phenomena has now been scientifically validated and several studies in the United States have demonstrated that if your pain centralises on performing the exercises, your chances of rapid and complete recovery are excellent. **Conversely, activities or positions which cause the pain to move away from the low back and perhaps increase in the buttock or leg are the wrong activities or incorrect positions.**

If your low back pain is of such intensity that you can only move around with difficulty and cannot find a position to lie comfortably in bed, your approach to the exercises should be cautious and unhurried.

On commencing any of the exercises you may experience an increase in pain. **This initial pain increase is common and can be expected.** As you continue to practice the pain should quickly diminish, at least to its former level. **This usually occurs during the first exercise session** and should then be followed by centralisation of pain. Once the pain no longer spreads outwards and is felt in the midline only, the intensity of the pain will decrease rapidly over a period of two to three days, and in anything from one to three or four weeks the pain should disappear entirely. If, following an initial pain increase, the pain continues to increase in intensity or spreads

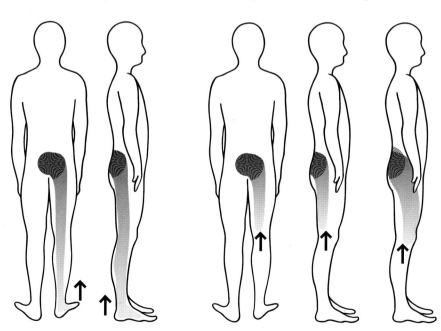

to places further away from the spine, you should stop exercising and seek advice. In other words, do not continue with any of the exercises **if your symptoms are much worse immediately after exercising and remain worse the next day;** or if, during exercising, symptoms are **produced or increased in the leg below the knee**.

If your symptoms have been present rather continuously for many weeks or months, you should not expect to be painfree in two to three days. The response will be slower but, if you are doing the correct exercises, it will only be a matter of ten to fourteen days before improvement begins.

When commencing this exercise programme you should stop any other exercises that you may have been shown elsewhere or happen to do regularly - for example, for fitness or sport. If you want to continue with exercises other than those described in this book for low back problems, you should wait until your pains have completely subsided.

New pains may develop as the result of performing movements your body is not used to and, provided you continue with the exercises, they will wear off in a few days. I always suspect that if my patients have not complained of new pains in different places, they have not been exercising adequately or they have not been putting enough effort into correcting their posture. Both of these situations, new exercises or new postures, should cause temporary new pains.

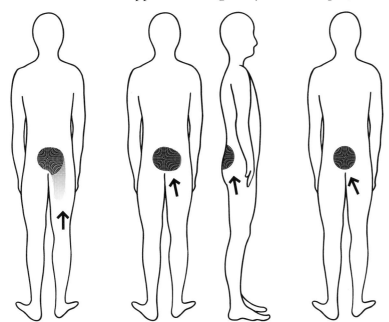

Fig 4.0 Progressive centralisation of pain indicates suitability of exercise programme

EXERCISE 1

Lying Face Down

Lie face down with your arms beside your body and your head turned to one side (*Fig.4:1*). Stay in this position, take a few deep breaths and then relax completely for two or three minutes. You must make a conscious effort to remove all tension from the muscles in your low back: without this complete relaxation there is no chance of eliminating any distortion that may be present in the joint.

This exercise is used mainly in the treatment of acute back pain and is one of the *first-aid* exercises. It should be done once at the beginning of each exercise session, and the sessions are to be spread evenly six to eight times throughout the day. This means that you should repeat the sessions about every two hours. In addition, you may lie face down whenever you are resting.

This exercise is performed in preparation for Exercise 2.

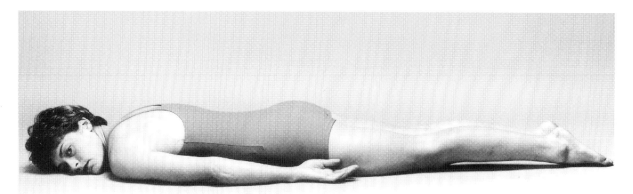

Fig 4.1

EXERCISE 2
Lying Face Down in Extension

Remain face down (*Fig.4:2a*). Place your elbows under your shoulders so that you lean on your forearms (*Fig.4:2b*). During this exercise (as with Exercise 1) you should commence by taking a few deep breaths and then allow the muscles in the low back to relax completely. You should remain in this position for two to three minutes.

Exercise 2 is used mainly in the treatment of severe low back pain and is one of the *first-aid* exercises. It should always follow Exercise 1 and is to be performed once per session.

Should you experience severe and increasing pain on attempting this exercise, there are certain measures to be taken before you can continue exercising. These are discussed in the next chapter under *No Response or Benefit*.

This exercise is performed in preparation for Exercise 3.

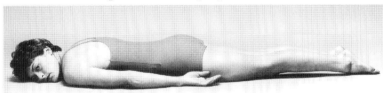

Fig 4.2a

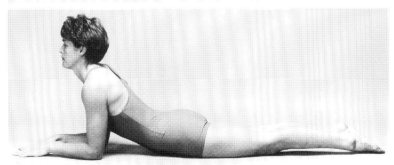

Fig 4.2b

EXERCISE 3

Extension in Lying

Remain face down (*Fig.4:3a*). Place your hands under your shoulders in the press-up position (*Fig.4:3b*). Now you are ready to commence Exercise 3.

Straighten your elbows and push the top half of your body up as far as pain permits (*Fig.4:3c*). It is important that you completely relax the pelvis, hips and legs as you do this. **Keep your pelvis, hips and legs hanging limp and allow your low back to sag.** Once you have maintained this position for a second or two, you should lower yourself to the starting position. Each time you repeat this movement cycle you should try to raise your upper body a little higher, so that in the end your back is extended as much as possible with your arms as straight as possible (Fig.4:3d). Once your arms are straight, remember to hold the *sag* for a second or two as this is a most important part of the exercise. The *sag* may be maintained for longer than one or two seconds if you feel the pain is reducing or centralising.

This is the most useful and effective first-aid procedure in the treatment of acute low back pain. The exercise can also be used to treat stiffness of the low back, and to prevent low back pain from recurring once you are fully recovered. When used in the treatment of either pain or stiffness, the exercise should be performed ten times per session and the sessions are to be spread evenly six to eight times throughout the day.

Should you not respond or have increasing pain on attempting this exercise, there are certain measures to be taken before you can continue exercising. These are discussed in the next chapter under "No Response or Benefit". Go to page 59 now.

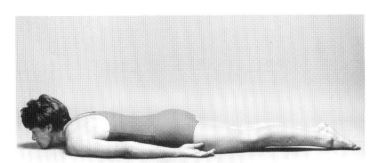

Fig 4.3a

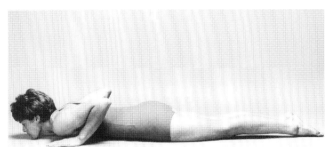

Fig 4.3b

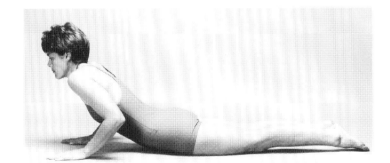

Fig 4.3c

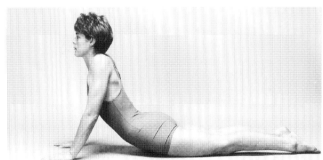

Fig 4.3d

4

EXERCISE 4

Extension in Standing

Stand upright with your feet slightly apart. Place your hands in the small of your back with the fingers pointing backwards (*Fig.4:4a*). You are now ready to commence Exercise 4.

Bend your trunk backwards at the waist **as far as you can**, using your hands as a fulcrum (*Fig.4:4b*). It is important that you **keep the knees straight** as you do this. Once you have maintained this position for a second or two, you should return to the starting position. Each time you repeat this movement cycle, you should try to bend backwards a little further so that in the end you have reached the maximum possible degree of extension.

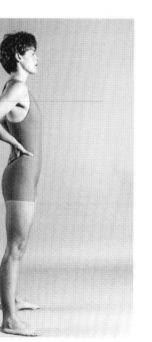

Fig 4.4a

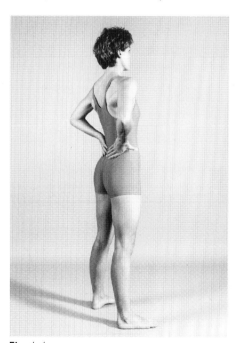

Fig 4.4a

When you are in acute pain, this exercise may replace Exercise 3 should circumstances prevent you from exercising in the lying position. This exercise, however, is not as effective as Exercise 3.

Once you are fully recovered and no longer have low back pain, this exercise is **your main tool in the prevention of further low back problems**. As a preventive measure, repeat the exercise every once in a while whenever you find yourself working in a forward bent position. Perform the exercise **before** pain appears.

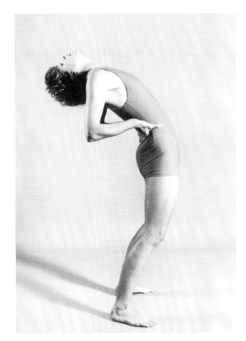

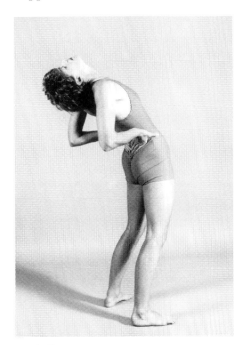

Fig 4.4b

Fig 4.4b

EXERCISE 5

Flexion in Lying

Lie on your back with your knees bent and your feet flat on the floor or bed (*Fig.4:5a*). You are now ready to commence Exercise 5.

Bring both knees up towards your chest (*Fig.4:5b*). Place both hands around your knees and gently but firmly pull the knees as close to the chest as pain permits (*Fig.4:5c*). Once you have maintained this position for a second or two you should lower the legs and return to the starting position. It is important that you **do not raise your head** as you perform this exercise, or **straighten your legs as you lower them**. Each time you repeat this movement cycle you should try to pull your knees a little closer to the chest so that in the end you have reached the maximum possible degree of flexion. At this stage your knees may touch the chest.

This exercise is used in the treatment of stiffness in the low back which may have developed since your injury or pain began. While damaged tissues may have now healed, they may also have shortened and become less flexible: it is now necessary to restore their elasticity and full function by performing flexion exercises. These exercises should be commenced with caution. In the beginning you must do only five or six repetitions per session, and the sessions are to be repeated three to four times per day. As you have probably realised, this exercise eliminates the lordosis once the knees are bent to the chest, so in order to rectify any distortion that may result, **flexion exercises must always be followed by a session of Exercise 3 - Extension in Lying**.

You may stop performing Exercise 5 when you can readily pull the knees to the chest without producing tightness or pain. You may then progress to Exercise 6.

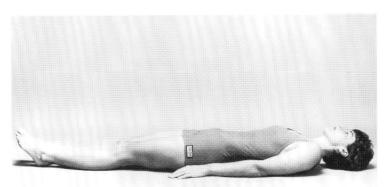

Fig 4.5

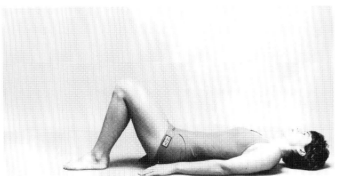

Fig 4.5a

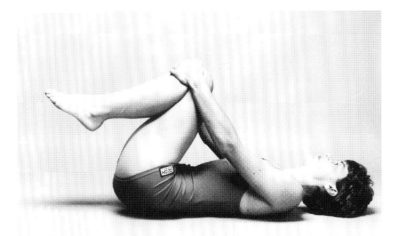

Fig 4.5b

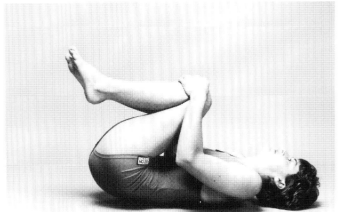

Fig 4.5c

EXERCISE 6

Flexion in Sitting

Sit on the edge of a steady chair with your knees and feet well apart and let your hands rest between your legs (*Fig.4:6a*). You are now ready to start Exercise 6.

Bend your trunk forwards and touch the floor with your hands (*Fig.4:6b*). Return immediately to the starting position. Each time your repeat this movement cycle, you must try to bend down a little further so that in the end you have reached the maximum possible degree of flexion and your head is as close as possible to the floor. The exercise can be made more effective by holding on to your ankles with your hands and pulling yourself down further (*Fig.4:6c* and *Fig.4:6d*).

Exercise 6 should only be commenced after the completion of one week of practice of Exercise 5, whether Exercise 5 has been successful or not in reducing your stiffness or pain. In the beginning you must do only five or six repetitions per session; the sessions are to be repeated three to four times per day and **must always be followed by Exercise 3.**

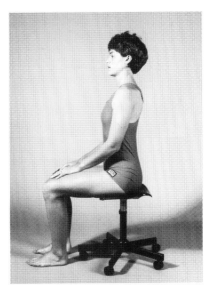

Fig 4.6a

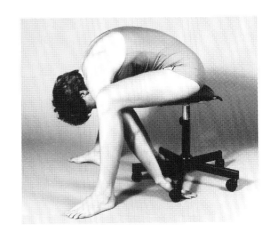

Fig 4.6b

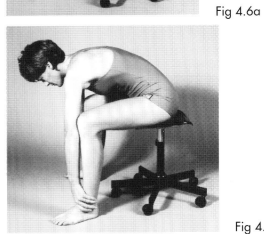

Fig 4.6c

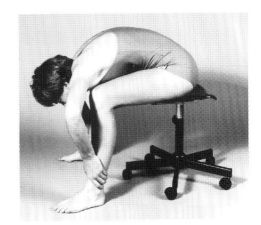

Fig 4.6d

4

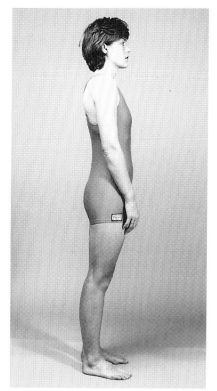

Fig 4.7a

EXERCISE 7

Flexion in Standing

Stand upright with your feet well apart. Allow your arms to hang loosely by your side.(*Fig.4:7a*) You are now ready to commence Exercise 7.

Bend forward and run your fingers down your legs as far as you can comfortably reach. (*Fig.4:7b*) Return immediately to the upright standing position. Each time your repeat this movement cycle, you must try to bend down a little further so that in the end you have reached the maximum possible degree of flexion and your finger tips are as close as possible to the floor.

Exercise 7 should only be commenced after the completion of two weeks of practice of Exercise 6, whether Exercise 6 has been successful or not in reducing your stiffness or pain. In the beginning you must do only five or six repetitions per session; the sessions are to be repeated once or twice per day **and must always be followed by Exercise 3.** For a period of three months from the time you have become pain free, Exercise 7 must never be performed in the first four hours of your day.

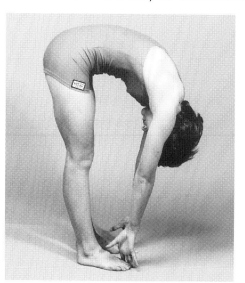

Fig 4.7b

CHAPTER 5

5

WHEN TO APPLY THE EXERCISES

You have probably experienced several acute or severe episodes of back pain in the past. You probably already know that the pain will pass off in time. What can you do to accelerate recovery? This section of the book is aimed at assisting you make a more rapid recovery. By learning from this experience you actually acquire a better insight into the steps you must take in the future if trouble strikes again. Yes, it can happen again; because when you feel good, you, like all others with the same problem, tend to forget the precautions you should take. The main thing is to learn how the manoeuvres described here affect your particular back problem.

WHEN YOU ARE IN SIGNIFICANT PAIN

A severe, acute attack of low back pain will cause pain that is felt at all times regardless of the position adopted or the movements being performed. It is made much worse by sitting or rising from sitting and by bending forwards. If the pain is also much worse on attempting to stand or walk and if you are unable to straighten up fully, it may not be possible for you to function and bed rest is the only alternative.

Recent research tells us that bed rest is not the best option for the treatment of acute and severe back pain and should be given for no more than two days. Those involved in that particular study, however, will perhaps alter that view if they ever personally experience a severe bout of the problem.

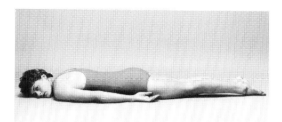

Exercise 1

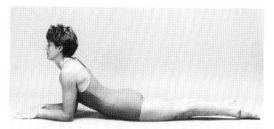

Exercise 2

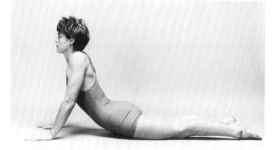

Exercise 3   Fig 5.1

In my experience, there are many patients in severe pain who require longer than two days of bed rest before ambulation is possible. Nevertheless, early activity, exercise and movement is desirable for those forced to seek bed rest, and a determined effort to stand upright should be attempted at an opportune time at least once each day.

You may commence the exercise programme during this period of bed rest provided you can lie face down for short periods. You should perform Exercises 1 through to 3 - Lying Face Down, Lying Face Down in Extension, and Extension in Lying (*Fig. 5:1*). **These exercises are first-aid for low back pain.** Immediately following the exercises, you should roll on to your back and insert the roll described on page 34 under the heading of *Correction of Surface*. This will maintain your back in the correct position during the period of bed rest.

You should seek advice from your family physician if your back pain is of such severity that it is impossible to perform any of the exercises or if your pain is becoming intolerable. Certain medications such as aspirin and nonsteroidal anti-inflammatory drugs (NSAIDS) may be necessary to provide some respite from pain. Both these drugs have been found to be the most useful for alleviation of acute back pain and have fewer side effects than some other commonly prescribed medications. Both have been recommended by the United States Federal Government Agency for Health Care Policy and Research.

If the pain is not severe enough to force you to rest in bed and if you are able to continue with some of your daily activities in spite of your pain, you should perform Exercises 1 through to 3 - Lying Face Down, Lying Face Down in Extension, and Extension in Lying.

The aim in performing Exercises 1 to 3 is to restore the lordosis to the fullest extent possible; then we must maintain it by careful attention to posture and movements at all times during the first week. You should avoid all rounded postures such as occur with bending or sitting slouched, and in fact you should sit as little as possible. Thus by avoiding flexion, the cause of any further distortion within the joint is removed, allowing healing to occur. (Remember the example of the finger?)

When commencing Exercise 3 you may initially experience an increase of pain in the low back; but with the repetition of the exercise, the pain should gradually reduce so that there is significant improvement by the time you have completed a few sessions. The pain may also become more localised in the centre of the back. This is desirable, as is any movement of pain from the legs and buttocks towards the middle of the back. In the end, the pain should disappear and be replaced by a feeling of strain or stiffness.

If your pain does not reduce or improve with these exercises please immediately read *No Response or Benefit*, page 59.

As soon as you feel considerably better and no longer have constant pain - perhaps a day or two after you have commenced exercising - you may stop Exercises 1 and 2, but you should continue Exercise 3 and add Exercise 4 - Extension in Standing.

About this time you should slowly introduce the slouch-overcorrect procedure, for you must now learn to sit correctly and maintain the lordosis just short of its maximum. As a rule, the pain will decrease as the lordosis increases and you will have no pain once you maintain the correct sitting posture. Pain will readily recur should you forget your posture and lose that vital hollow in your low back. Exercise 4 should be done whenever circumstances prevent the performance of Exercise 3: at regular intervals during sitting and working in a stooped position; and before and after lifting as well as during repeated lifting. The slouch-overcorrect procedure must be done two or three times per day until you are familiar with the correct sitting posture.

Once you no longer have acute pain, you should continue the exercise programme as outlined for *When Acute Pain Has Subsided*.

WHEN ACUTE PAIN HAS SUBSIDED

For the past few days you have been doing Exercises 1 to 4 and have been maintaining a lordosis at all times. Once the distortion in the joints has reduced and any damaged tissue healed it will be necessary to restore your flexibility and recover your normal function. This is achieved by performing flexion exercises, which must be carried out in such a way that no further damage or tearing occurs within the recently healed soft tissues. The risks of further damage are much less when the low back is rounded in the lying position than in standing. Therefore you must now perform Exercise 5 - Flexion in Lying.

Fig 5.2

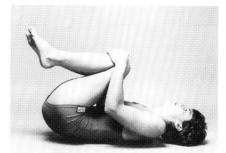

Exercise 5 - to be followed by . . .

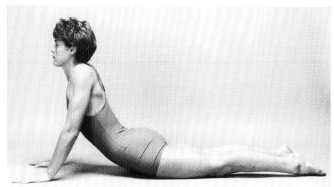

Exercise 3   Fig 5.2

Exercise 5 should be commenced when you have recovered from an acute episode of low back pain and have been painfree for two to three weeks, even though you may still feel stiffness on bending forwards. Exercise 5 may also be necessary should you have improved significantly with Exercises 1 to 4 but after two to three weeks still experience a small amount of pain in the centre of the back, which does not seem to disappear.

It is not uncommon for some central, midline, low back pain to be produced when starting with flexion in lying. An initial pain which wears off gradually with repetition of the exercise is acceptable, it means that shortened structures are being stretched effectively. However, if flexion in lying produces pain which increases with each repetition, you should stop. In this case it is either too soon to start flexion or the exercise is not suitable for your condition.

When you can touch your chest with the knees easily and without discomfort, you have regained full movement., You may now stop Exercise 5, and commence Exercise 6-(Fig.5.3). After two to three weeks, Exercise 6 should cause no tightness or discomfort and once you have reached this point you may add Exercise 7 to your programme-(Fig.5.4). Exercise 7 should be carried out at the end of the day once or twice a week to ensure that all the soft tissues in the back remain extensible.After completing Exercise 6 and 7 you should follow the guidelines given to prevent recurrence of low back problems and continue with the exercise programme as outlined for *When You Have No Pain Or Stiffness.*

IMPORTANT – Exercises 5, 6 and 7 should always be followed by Exercise 3 – Extension in Lying-(*Fig.5.2*). In this way you can rectify any distortion that could develop from Exercise 5, 6 or 7.

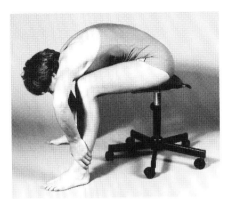

Exercise 6   Fig 5.3

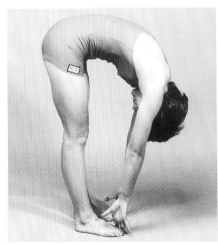

Exercise 7   Fig 5.4

WHEN YOU HAVE NO PAIN OR STIFFNESS

Many people with low back problems have lengthy spells in which they experience little or no pain. If, in the past or recently, you have had one or more episodes of low back pain, you should start or continue the exercise programme even though you may be painfree at the moment. However, in this situation it is not necessary to do all the exercises nor is it necessary to exercise every two hours.

To prevent recurrence of low back problems you should:

1. Perform Exercise 3 – Extension in Lying – on a regular basis, preferably in the morning and evening.

2. Perform Exercise 4 – Extension in Standing - at regular intervals whenever you are required to sit or bend forwards for long periods. You should also do Exercise 4 before and after heavy lifting and during repeated lifting, and whenever you feel minor strain developing in your low back.

3. Practice the slouch-overcorrect procedure whenever you are becoming negligent about the correct sitting posture.

4. Perform Exercise 7 once or twice a week to remain fully flexible.

5. Always use a lumbar roll in chairs which do not provide adequate support.

You should continue these exercises and adopt them as a regular part of your life. It is essential, however, that you do them **before the onset of pain.** Apart from exercising, it is even more important that you watch your posture at all times and never again let postural stresses be the cause of low back problems. The best exercises will have little or no effect if you constantly fall back into poor posture.

Thus, it is advisable to exercise in the manner described above for the rest of your life, but it is a necessity that you develop and maintain good postural habits. Remember, if you lose the lordosis for long periods at a time, you are risking recurrence of low back pain.

As it takes only one minute to perform one session of Exercise 3 and two minutes to complete one session of the slouch-overcorrect procedure, lack of time should never be used as an excuse for not being able to do these exercises.

NO RESPONSE OR BENEFIT

After exercising without any relief or benefit for three or four days, you may conclude that the exercises as performed are ineffectual. There are two main causes for lack of response or benefit from these exercises. A lack of response to these exercises is possible in some people when their pain is felt only to one side of the spine, or is felt much more to one side than the other. If your pain during the course of the day is felt only to one side, more to one side than the other, or if you feel pain more to one side as you perform Exercises 1, 2 or 3, you may need to modify your body position before commencing them.

To achieve this modification, you should:

1. Adopt the position to perform Exercise 1 and allow yourself to relax for a few minutes (Fig.5:5).
2. Remain face down and now shift your hips away from the painful side: that is, if your pain is usually more on the right side you must move your hips three or four inches to the left and once more completely relax for a few minutes (Fig.5:6)
3. While allowing the hips to remain off-centre, lean on the elbows as described in Exercise 2, and relax for a further three or four minutes (Fig.5:7)

5

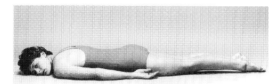

Fig 5.5   Step 1. Lie face down.

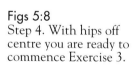

Figs 5.6
Step 2. Move your hips
away from pain.

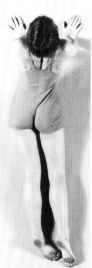

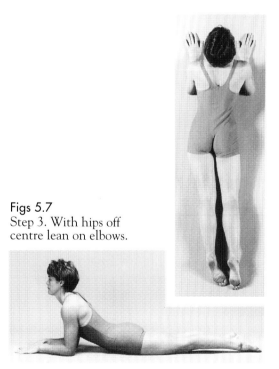

Figs 5.7
Step 3. With hips off
centre lean on elbows.

Figs 5:8
Step 4. With hips off
centre you are ready to
commence Exercise 3.

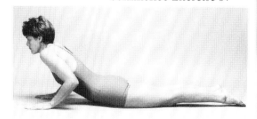

You are now ready to commence Exercise 3. With the hips still off-centre, complete one session of Exercise 3 (*Fig 5:8*) and then relax once more. You may need to repeat the exercise several times, but before commencing each session of ten you should ensure that the hips are still off-centre; remember, away from the painful side. Even with your hips in the off-centre position, you should try with each repetition to move higher and higher. You should reach the maximum amount of extension possible, at which time the arms should be completely straight.

For the next three or four days you should continue to perform Exercises 1, 2, and 3 from the modified starting position. The frequency of the exercise and the number of sessions per day should be the same as recommended in the section *When In Significant Pain*, page 53.

After a few days of practice, you may notice that the pain is distributed more evenly across the back or may have centralised. Once this occurs you may stop shifting the hips before exercising and continue exercises as recommended in the section *When in Significant Pain*, page 53. Occasionally, shifting the hips away from the painful side is sufficient to stop the pain completely.

The second cause for lack of response arises when Exercise 3 is performed without adequate fixation. Exercise 3 occasionally gives benefit for a few hours only, and then the pain returns. The effectiveness of Exercise 3 can be improved by holding the pelvis down using the hands of another person, or by constructing a simple device which can be improvised at home using an ironing board with a seat belt or strong leather strap

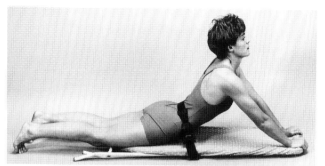

Fig 5.9 Added fixation

firmly around the waistline. This added fixation frequently makes the difference between the success or failure of the exercise. (*Fig.5:9*)

RECURRENCE

Irrespective of what you are doing or where you are, at the first sign of recurrence of low back pain you should immediately start the exercises which previously led to recovery and follow the instructions given to relieve acute pain. You should at once commence Exercise 4 – Extension in Standing. If this does not abolish your pain **within minutes**, you must quickly introduce Exercise 3 – Extension in Lying: the immediate performance of Exercise 3 can so often prevent the onset of a disabling attack. If your pain is already too severe to tolerate these exercises, you should commence with Exercises 1 and 2 – Lying Face Down, and Lying Face Down in Extension.

Finally, if you have one-sided symptoms which do not centralise with the exercises recommended so far, you should shift your hips away from the painful side before commencing the exercises and hold your hips in the off-centre position while you exercise. In addition to the exercises, you must pay extra attention to your posture and maintain the lordosis as much as possible.

If this episode of low back pain seems to be different from previous occasions and if your pain persists despite the fact that you closely follow the instructions, you should seek advice from a health professional or Member or Associate of the McKenzie Institute.

To obtain the names of Credentialed Members or Associates of the McKenzie Institute, see the Directory included at the back of the book.

CHAPTER 6

INSTRUCTIONS FOR PEOPLE WITH ACUTE LOW BACK PAIN

IMMEDIATELY COMMENCE THE SELF-TREATMENT EXERCISES

The simple rule is that if bending forwards has been the cause of overstretching, bending backwards should rectify this problem and reduce any resultant distortion. You must restore the lordosis slowly and with caution, never quickly or with jerky movements. You must allow some time for the distorted joint to regain its normal shape and position: a sudden or violent movement may retard this process, increase the strain in and around the affected joint, and thus result in an increase of low back pain.

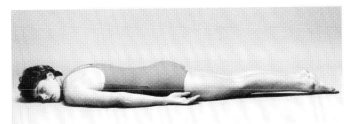

Exercise 1

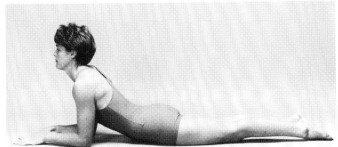

Exercise 2

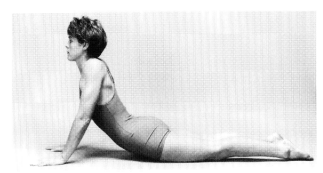

Exercise 3

6

Remember when commencing the exercises, some increase of midline low back pain can be expected. Some exercises will only be effective when you actually move into the pain while exercising. You should feel some pain when doing these exercises, but you should never have a lasting increase in pain which remains present the following day.

When in acute pain you must, apart from exercising, make certain adjustments in your daily activities. These adjustments form a very important aspect of self-treatment. If you do not follow the instructions given below, you will unnecessarily delay the healing process. **This is entirely your responsibility.**

Maintain your lumbar lordosis at all times. Slouched sitting and bending forwards as in touching the toes will only increase the pressure in the joints, stretch and weaken the supporting structures, and lead to further damage in the low back. If you slouch you will have discomfort and pain. **Good posture is the key to spinal comfort.**

Sit as little as possible, and then for short periods only. If you must sit, choose a firm high chair with a straight back, make sure that you have an adequate lordosis, and use a lumbar roll to support the low back. Avoid sitting on a low, soft couch with the legs straight out in front as in sitting up in bed or in the bath; both these situations force you to lose the lordosis.

When getting up from the sitting position, you should attempt to maintain the lordosis: move to the front of the seat, stand up by straightening the legs and avoid bending forwards at the waist.

Drive the car as little as possible, it is better to be a passenger than to drive yourself. If you must drive, your seat should be far enough back from the steering wheel to allow you to drive with your arms relatively straight. With the arms straight, your upper body is held back and you are prevented from slouching; this allows full benefit to be obtained from the lumbar roll, which should always be used when driving. Avoid activities which require bending forwards or stooping. Many activities can be modified adequately to enable maintenance of the lordosis. It is possible to maintain the correct posture when vacuuming in the standing position; it is also possible to maintain a correct lordosis by going down on all fours when gardening, making beds, etc.

If you have acute low back pain, you should not lift at all. If you must lift, you should avoid objects that are awkward to handle or heavier than thirty pounds (15 kg). At all times you must use the correct lifting technique.

If you are uncomfortable at night, you may benefit from a supportive roll around your waist. For most people, it is recommended that the mattress should not be too hard but well-supported by a firm base. If your bed sags, slats or a sheet of plywood between mattress and base will straighten it, or else you can have the mattress placed on the floor.

When getting up from lying, you should keep your back in lordosis: turn on one side, draw both knees up, drop the feet over the edge of the bed, raise yourself to the sitting position by pushing your upper body up with your hands, and avoid bending forwards at the waist. Stand up from sitting as described before.

Avoid coughing and sneezing while you are sitting or bending forwards. You should stand and bend backwards if you are forced to cough or sneeze.

Avoid those positions and movements which initially caused your problems. You must allow some time for healing to take place.

CHAPTER 7

SPECIAL SITUATIONS

TREATMENT BY "REPEX"

Although the system of self-treatment that I have developed is effective for a large number of patients, the success of the method is sometimes limited because of various factors which may prevent the patient from performing the required movements.

Fatigue is probably the most commonly encountered limiting factor. Patients find that they are unable to continue exercising because their arms have become too tired. This is particularly frustrating for the patient whose pain is improving with the exercises but who cannot continue with them because of fatigue.

Some patients are unable to relax sufficiently when performing the push-up exercise. For the exercise to be effective, it is vital that relaxation be obtained in the lower back.

Some patients, especially the elderly, may have shoulder, elbow or wrist complaints which prevent them performing the key exercises.

Patients with certain disorders can have such restricted movement that the self-treatment exercises are impossible to perform.

To overcome these difficulties, in 1986 I engaged an engineer to develop a machine to provide controlled doses of specific repeated movements to the lower back.

The machine, named "REPEX", can continuously move the lower back many hundreds of times if necessary, without the patient having to exert him or herself at all.

(**REPEX** stands for **R**epeated **E**ndrange **P**assive **EX**ercise)

This form of treatment known as CPM, or continuous passive motion, has been found to provide better quality healing and more rapid recovery when applied to other injured joints of the body. REPEX is the first such machine to provide CPM for mechanical low back disorders.

If you have not resolved your back problem already with the methods described in this book, it may well be that the REPEX could assist further. It is possible that REPEX could help with your problem, particularly if you get relief after each session of exercise but the relief does not last. In this case it may well be that an increased number of movements may be all that is required to obtain lasting relief.

Treatment by REPEX requires specialist expertise and is available only through Credentialed Members or Associates of the McKenzie Institute.

To obtain the names of Credentialed Members or Associates of the McKenzie Institute, see the Directory included at the back of the book.

LOW BACK PAIN IN PREGNANCY

Both during and after pregnancy women are subjected to altered mechanical stresses which affect the low back and frequently result in low back problems. As the new infant develops in the mother's womb, two simple changes take place which influence her posture.

Firstly, there is the gradually increasing bulk and weight of the developing infant. In order to maintain balance during standing and walking, the mother must lean further backwards to counterbalance her altered weight distribution. The result of this postural adjustment is an increase in lordosis. In the final weeks

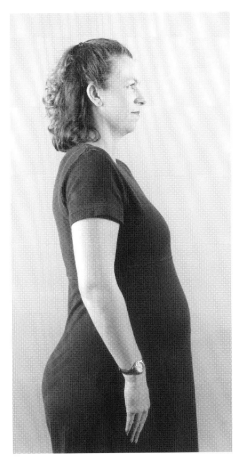

Fig 7.0 Low back pain in Pregnancy

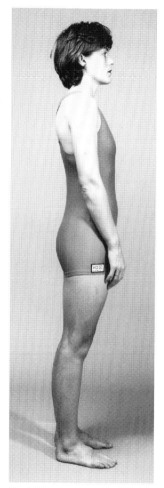

Fig 7.1

of pregnancy the lordosis may become excessive and this may lead to overstretching of the tissues surrounding the joints of the low back (*Fig.7*).

Secondly, to prepare the body for the impending delivery of the baby, the joints of the pelvis and lower back are made more flexible and elastic by a natural increase of certain hormones. This greater elasticity means that the joints involved become more lax and are easily overstretched when subjected to mechanical strains.

After the child is born the mother is often too busy to care for herself properly, and sometimes the postural fault which has developed during pregnancy remains present for the rest of her life.

If your back problems commenced during or after pregnancy, it is likely that your lordosis has become excessive and your problems are caused mainly by postural stresses. If this is the case, the extension exercises recommended for the majority of people with low back pain are unsuitable for you at the present time, and you should concentrate mainly on correction of the standing posture (*Fig.7:1*). Problems caused by postural stresses are always resolved by postural correction. For one week you must watch your posture very closely. At all times you should maintain the correct posture, not only during standing but also while walking. You must **stand tall and walk tall** and not allow yourself to slouch. If after one week of postural correction the pain has disappeared or reduced considerably, faulty posture is to be blamed for your back problems.

If your back problems commenced during or after pregnancy and **you feel worse when standing and walking but much better when sitting**, extension exercises again are not suitable for you. Now you should, in addition to the postural correction in standing and

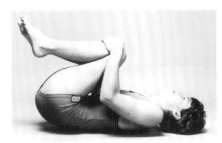

Fig 7.2

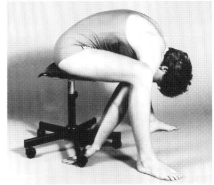

Fig 7.2a

walking, perform flexion exercises and self-treatment consisting of excises 5 and 6 – Flexion in Lying, and Flexion in Sitting (*Fig.7:2*) and(*Fig.7:2a*). During the first week you should perform Exercise 5 at regular intervals - that is, ten times per session and six to eight sessions per day. When you have improved to some extent with this procedure, you should add Exercise 6 in the second week. Exercise 6 must follow Exercise 5 and should be done with the same frequency. **Flexion exercises performed to relieve back pain appearing during pregnancy should not be followed by extension in lying.** Once you are completely painfree, you may stop Exercise 5. In order to prevent recurrence of low back problems you should continue Exercise 6 twice per day, preferably in the morning and evening. At all times you should maintain good postural habits, but a lumbar roll should not be used in your case.

If you are uncertain as to which of these two categories you belong, or if you do not respond to the flexion exercises, you should consult a Credentialed Member or Associate of the McKenzie Institute.

LOW BACK PAIN IN ATHLETES

After forty-five years of practice, I have come to the conclusion that low back problems occurring in athletes require more than the usual amount of attention. The symptoms of low back pain occurring in athletes can often behave in an extremely mystifying and confusing fashion. A combination of several factors add to this confusion.

Firstly, athletes are highly motivated to participate in their treatment, and sometimes carry to excess the advice given to them in an attempt to speed recovery. This over-exuberant participation in the rehabilitation of their back problem very often delays rather than accelerates the healing process.

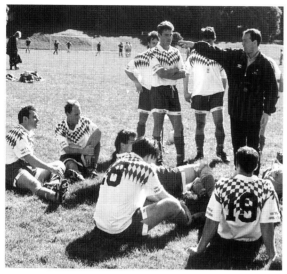

Fig 7.3 Slouched positions

A second point to be noted is that the athlete or sportsman's enthusiasm to participate in their favourite pastime or sport leads them to return to full participation, often long before sufficient time has passed to allow for complete healing.

The third and certainly the most common source of confusion can stem from the frequent belief of athletes that the sole cause of their problem lies in their frequent participation in a particular sporting activity. Subsequently, this belief is reinforced by a health provider who all too often comes to the same conclusion. It is not difficult to reach this conclusion, for probably three out of five athletes who experience low back pain state that their pain appears after they have participated in sport or indulged in some equally vigorous activity.

The belief that pain appearing shortly after activity must be caused by the activity itself is widespread and understandable but unfortunately frequently mistaken.

The true cause of pain in these individuals is frequently the adoption of a slouched position following the thorough exercising of their joints (*Fig.7:3*). After exertion we usually sit down and relax: as we are tired, the relaxed sitting posture is adopted almost immediately. In other words, after vigorous exercising we collapse in a heap and slouch badly. Joints of the spine during the process of vigorous exercise are moved rapidly in many directions over an extended period of time. This process causes a thorough stretching in all directions of the soft tissues surrounding the joints. In addition, the fluid gel content of the spinal discs is loosened, and it seems that distortion or displacement can occur if an exercised joint is subsequently placed in an extreme posture. This is so often the cause of back pain in athletes and can be proven rather easily as shall be explained.

If low back pain has in fact occurred as a result of participation in a sport, then recommending rest from activity would be appropriate advice. However, if the pain has appeared after the activity has been completed and has occurred as a result of adopting a slouched sitting posture, such advice would be entirely inappropriate. To advise an athlete to cease participation in his favourite pastime can have serious consequences both emotional and physical.

If you are an athlete or if you participate in vigorous activities and have recently developed low back pain, it is necessary to expose the true cause of this problem in order to treat your condition correctly and successfully: we must determine whether your pain appeared **during** the particular activity or whether it developed **afterwards**. If the pain appeared during the activity itself, then your sport may well be the cause of the present problems. You may remember something which happened at the time of the activity and can describe what you felt at that moment: but a very large number of people who have back pain and participate in sport, never feel discomfort or pain while they are participating or competing, their pain appears after the activity.

It is easy to determine if your low back problems are the result of slouched sitting. From now on, **immediately after activity**, you should watch your posture closely and sit correctly with the low back in moderate lordosis supported by a lumbar roll (*Fig.7:4* and *Fig.7:4a*). For example, if you have completed a few sets of tennis, if you have finished a round of golf, or competed in a football game, you must not then sink into a comfortable lounge chair or slouch in the car when you drive home (fig.7:5). You must sit correctly with posture maintained meticulously. Should no pain eventuate as a result of this extra postural care, the answer to your problem is clear and the responsibility for preventing further trouble is entirely your own.

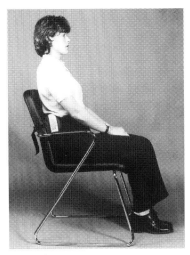

Fig 7.4

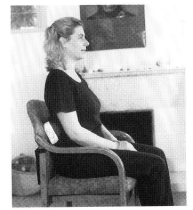

Fig 7.4a

If you fall into the group of people who **develop pain only after activity,** it is undesirable for you to begin the **exercises** at the same time as commencing the postural correction. If the exercises are performed in conjunction with postural correction, it is impossible to determine from which source the improvement was derived.

If your pain continues to appear after activity in spite of correcting your posture, it is possible that you have weakened or damaged some of the soft tissues in your low back. If this is the case, now is the time to commence self-treatment and you should perform Exercises 3 and 4 – Extension in Lying and Extension in Standing – on a regular basis.

Poor posture is often seen in athletes during intervals of non-participation: for example when waiting their turn to high jump, throw the discus or bat at baseball. It is necessary to maintain good posture during these intervals as well as after completion of the activity.

If your pain appears regularly **while** running or jogging, you should commence the self-treatment programme as outlined earlier under the heading *When In Acute Pain.* You should also seek advice regarding the type of footwear you use, the surface you run on and, possibly, your running technique. If your problems persist despite following the advice, you may need special treatment.

LOW BACK PAIN IN THE ELDERLY

It is now known that acute low back pain tends to occur less once we pass the age of 55; so if you are over 55 or thereabouts, you may notice that you experience a more persistent ache in the low back but no longer have the acute and severe episodes that affected you in your more active and vigorous days. Nevertheless, this aching can cause

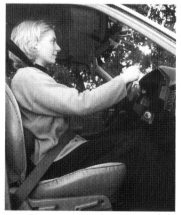

Fig 7.5

significant problems, especially if you are forced to reduce activity. The human body thrives on activity and decays with prolonged inactivity. It is undesirable for any of us, irrespective of age, to reduce our levels of activity. Only if reduced activity is forced upon us by significant health related problems, should we exercise less.

You may also be told that you have degenerative changes in your back or that you have arthritis and will *just have to live with it*. While it may be true that your back has worn somewhat with ageing, it is certainly not true that *you will just have to live with it*. It has been found that many people who have joints in their spines that are worn with age, have never had back pain and we now know that the wearing in itself is not a cause of pain.

It is my experience that there are few persons who will not derive some benefit from the postural advice or the exercises, or both. Every older person should carry out the advice regarding the correction of the sitting, standing, and lying postures.

Not all of you in the older group will be able to carry out all the exercises as advised, but you should **all** try. I have found that age is not necessarily a barrier to the successful application of the exercises and, although there are some who may not succeed because of weakness or disability, most will be able to advance at least part way through the recommended programme.

My advice to you is to start by perhaps reducing the number of exercises to be performed at each session and to perform fewer sessions during the day. Do not hurry the process and always rest adequately after completing the exercises - properly supported in the correct position, of course!

OSTEOPOROSIS

From middle age many women are affected by a disorder called osteoporosis. This is essentially a mineral deficiency disorder. During and after menopause, there is a significant and continuing deficiency in calcium replacement which must in many cases be supplemented with calcium tablets on a regular basis. As a consequence of calcium deficiency there is a weakening of bone structure resulting in a slow but progressive reduction in bone height. This in turn allows the postures of those affected to become extremely rounded especially in the mid or thoracic part of the spine.

In persons affected by this disorder there are risks of fractures occurring without any significant forces being applied to the bones of the vertebrae. Research conducted at the Mayo Clinic in the United States has demonstrated that extension exercises

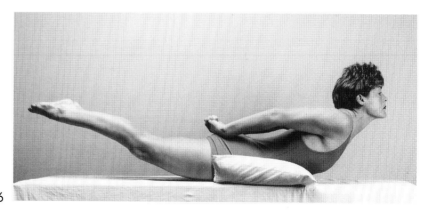

Fig 7.6

performed regularly (*Fig.7:6*) had significantly reduced the number of compression fractures in the group exercising in this manner. A similar group exercising differently and a group not exercising at all had significantly more fractures when examined at least one year later. This study suggests that women from perhaps the age of forty onwards, should practice this exercise as described on a regular basis. My own recommendation would be that the exercise should be performed fifteen to twenty times, four or five times per week. If you are uncertain regarding this advice, discuss the matter with your doctor before commencing the programme. Should you have difficulties with the exercises for one reason or another, you should consult a manipulative therapist who will show you means of modifying the exercise without necessarily reducing its effectiveness.

The muscles strengthened by performing the exercises recommended by the Mayo Clinic study, are also the muscles responsible for holding you upright and it is probable that maintaining good posture at all times will assist in the strengthening process. This may also reduce the likelihood of small fractures occurring.

CHAPTER 8

COMMON REMEDIES AND SOLUTIONS

MEDICINES AND DRUGS

As mentioned earlier in this book, most of the common back pains we experience are mechanical in origin and therefore are affected only by drugs and medication with pain relieving capabilities. There are no medicines or drugs capable of removing the causes of our common backaches and pains. Therefore, medication should only be taken when your pains are severe or when you must find relief.

Certain medications such as aspirin and non-steroidal anti-inflammatory drugs (NSAIDS) have been found to be the most useful for alleviation of acute back pain and have fewer side effects than some other commonly prescribed medications. Both have been recommended by the US Federal Government Agency for Health Care Policy and Research.

BEDREST

When your back pain is so severe that bed rest is required, you should restrict this period of rest if at all possible, to two or three days.

A recent study conducted in the United States demonstrated that those patients resting in bed for two days recovered as well as those remaining in bed for seven days. However, those patients remaining ambulant and moving were able to go back to work sooner than those who rested for either two or seven days. Nevertheless, I have seen many patients who could still not arise from bed after ten days.

ACUPUNCTURE

Acupuncture is able to relieve pain and when all else has failed, is well worth a trial. You should be aware, however, that like taking medication you can obtain relief from acupuncture but acupuncture itself does not correct the underlying mechanical problem.

CHIROPRACTIC AND OSTEOPATHY

In the past, the treatment of back and neck problems by adjustment or manipulation of the spine was considered one of the most popular forms of treatment and it was demonstrated by chiropractors and osteopaths in the first half of the century that a short-term benefit could be obtained from this form of treatment. However, much research has now shown that from spinal manipulation or adjustment there are no long-term benefits and its use can create dependency.

A recent study by internationally renowned researchers from the University of Washington in the United States has shown that one month after completing treatment, patients taught the McKenzie method improved to the same degree as patients receiving manipulation by chiropractors. However, the patients receiving the McKenzie method had fewer treatments to achieve that improvement and 72% of them reported that in the event of recurrence they would manage their own problem. This has great significance for those patients with recurring problems.

About 80% of patients with common back problems can be taught the self-manipulation methods outlined in this book. The other 20% of the population are the only ones who will require any form of manipulative therapy.

I think it is important that people who are suffering from back pain are aware that spinal manipulation or adjustive treatments should

..

not be given to the whole population with back pain in order to deliver it to the few who really need it. Spinal manipulation should certainly not be used before self-treatment measures have proven unsuccessful.

Manipulative physiotherapists, chiropractors and osteopaths all dispense spinal manipulation or "adjustment". The techniques used by all three groups are similar. The theory and rationale for providing the procedures is completely different in all three groups.

Manipulative physiotherapists and chiropractors who are Members or Associates of the McKenzie Institute, are well versed in the entire range of mechanical treatments in use for back pain today, including manipulation. (See Directory)

Not all chiropractors use the procedures described in this book but several Chiropractic Colleges in the United States are now teaching the methods through Faculty of the McKenzie Institute International.

Non medically qualified osteopaths by virtue of their training are not yet eligible to attend the McKenzie Institute International Education Programme.

ELECTROTHERAPY

In 1995, the United States Federal Government Agency for Health Care Policy and Research published a list of recommendations to guide those health professionals involved in acute back care. Because there was no supportive scientific evidence, the Agency could not recommend various forms of heat, shortwave diathermy, and ultrasound, all of which are commonly used in the treatment of back pain.

You should be aware that these treatments provide no long-term benefit and do nothing to treat the underlying problem, nor is there any scientific evidence that they can accelerate healing.

BACK PAIN IN THE COMMUNITY

Low back pain is widespread throughout the world, both in western and eastern cultures. It has been estimated that by the year 2000 one billion people living on this planet will have experienced back pain of one sort or another.

So many things could be done to improve this situation. You as an individual should complain wherever you find inappropriate seating in public offices or buildings and on public transport. You should complain to your car dealer if the vehicle seats are inadequate: better still, look for another car!

When choosing lounge furniture (which is nearly always designed to cause or perpetuate back problems) you should persist until you find chairs which are properly designed. Management in furniture stores should be told in no uncertain terms that the seating they provide is poorly designed, where this is found to be the case.

There are few airlines providing seating which adequately supports the low back; this has serious consequences for some individuals who must fly over long distances for many hours at a time.

Office workers should demand seating which provides adequate lumbar support. There are many sophisticated and expensive office and secretarial chairs on the market which provide no support whatsoever.

Although poor seating design is a major contributing factor to the development of low back pain, another and more important factor is becoming increasingly evident. Where once our school physical education instructors were concerned with and corrected faulty posture in children, they now seem to be more interested in producing the best football team, the best high-jumper, and the fastest runner. Physical educationists in all parts of the world seem to no longer equip our children with the information that is so necessary if they are to care for their own physical needs during a lifetime on this planet. Spinal pain of postural origin would not occur if this basic education were given to individuals at an early age. Ask any twelve-year old child if he or she has been shown at school how to stand correctly, or how to sit correctly. The chances are that they will tell you they have never been shown either of these two basic and fundamental postures, nor have they been acquainted with the possible harmful consequences that may occur by neglecting them.

If these matters are of concern to you, a polite request could be made to your school administration or physical education instructors asking that postural physical education of children be made a priority. In addition, school furniture must come under scrutiny for it is difficult to find well designed seating in any school. Good postural habits must be instilled at an early age.

These are the steps that you as a concerned individual can take to assist in bringing about some of the changes that must occur if society is to grapple sensibly with this enormous problem, which in the United States in 1982 cost approximately 14 billion dollars in compensation, treatment, and rehabilitation.

CHAPTER 9

PANIC PAGE

IN CASE OF SUDDEN ONSET OF ACUTE PAIN
CARRY OUT THE FOLLOWING INSTRUCTIONS:

1 **IMMEDIATELY LIE FACE DOWN**
   If this is impossible because of pain intensity,
   go to bed.
   Attempt exercises next day.

2 **USE A ROLLED TOWEL OR A NIGHT ROLL
   AROUND YOUR WAIST WHEN RESTING IN
   BED.**

3 **PERFORM EXERCISES 1, 2 AND 3, TEN
   TIMES EVERY TWO HOURS.**

4 **IF THE PAIN IS MORE TO ONE SIDE AND
   NOT REDUCING, MOVE HIPS AWAY FROM
   THE PAINFUL SIDE AND DO EXERCISES 2
   AND 3.**

5 **REST AS MUCH AS POSSIBLE, CORRECTLY
   SUPPORTED.**

6 **DO NOT BEND FORWARD FOR 3-4 DAYS.**

7 **SIT PERFECTLY AT ALL TIMES - USE A
   LUMBAR ROLL.**

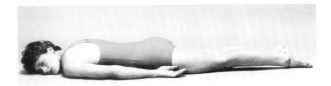

Exercise 1

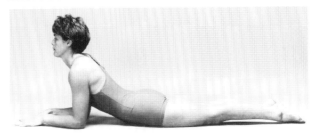

Exercise 2

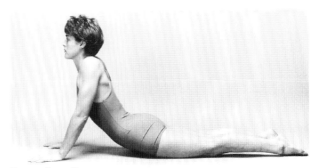

Exercise 3

WORLD DIRECTORY

If you wish to locate the address or telephone number of your nearest Credentialed Member or Associate of the McKenzie Institute, call:

Australia	**(02) 9743-3808**
Canada	**(905) 836-5206**
Denmark	**(42) 523-358**
Germany	**08367-1299**
The Netherlands	**(543) 517-492**
New Zealand	**(04) 293-6645**
Sweden	**(8)791-8887 (fax)**
Switzerland	**(81)723-7349 (fax)**
The United Kingdom	**(01993) 832-592**
The United States of America	**800 635-8380**

The McKenzie Institute International Spinal Therapy and Rehabilitation Centres have been established for the purposes of providing treatment programmes for patients with chronic and recurring back and neck problems.

The Institute works directly with referring physicians in formulating individualised ongoing self-treatment programmes.

If you would like more information about the Institute programmes, please contact one of the above numbers.

More help for
back and neck pain sufferers

Information Pack - Prevention and Self-Help

For an information pack on prevention and self-help treatments compiled by the National Back Pain Association please fill in the slip below and return to the Freepost address overleaf.

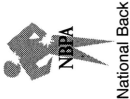

National Back
Pain Association

Name ....
(BLOCK CAPITALS)

Address ....

....

....

Postcode ....

McKenzie Back and Neck Supports

☐ Please send me further information on the McKenzie range of orthopaedic back and neck supports used in this book.

These supports are available by mail order from Procare Medipost, distributors of McKenzie self-help books and supports in Europe.

Materials requested will be sent only by post. You have our assurance **NO** personal or telephone sales calls will follow the completion of this request slip. Procare Medipost does not employ sales representatives.

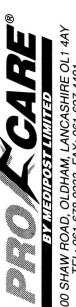

PRO CARE®
BY MEDIPOST LIMITED

100 SHAW ROAD, OLDHAM, LANCASHIRE OL1 4AY
TEL: 061-678 0233 FAX: 061-627 4401

Procare is a Trade Mark of Medipost

Pro-care Medipost Ltd
FREEPOST
100 Shaw Road
Oldham
Lancs.
OL1 4BR